FITTER
FASTER

FITTER FASTER

THE SMART WAY
TO GET IN SHAPE IN
JUST MINUTES A DAY

ROBERT J. DAVIS, PH.D.

with Brad Kolowich, Jr.

ᴬMACOM

American Management Association

New York * Atlanta * Brussels * Chicago * Mexico City * San Francisco
Shanghai * Tokyo * Toronto * Washington, DC

Bulk discounts available. For details visit:
www.amacombooks.org/go/specialsales
Or contact special sales:
Phone: 800-250-5308
Email: specialsls@amanet.org
View all the AMACOM titles at: www.amacombooks.org

American Management Association: www.amanet.org
This publication is designed to provide accurate and authoritative information in regard to the subject matter covered. It is sold with the understanding that the publisher is not engaged in rendering legal, accounting, or other professional service. If legal advice or other expert assistance is required, the services of a competent professional person should be sought.

Library of Congress data is available upon request.

ISBN: 9780814437711
EISBN: 9780814437728

About AMA

American Management Association (www.amanet.org) is a world leader in talent development, advancing the skills of individuals to drive business success. Our mission is to support the goals of individuals and organizations through a complete range of products and services, including classroom and virtual seminars, webcasts, webinars, podcasts, conferences, corporate and government solutions, business books, and research. AMA's approach to improving performance combines experiential learning—learning through doing—with opportunities for ongoing professional growth at every step of one's career journey.

10 9 8 7 6 5 4 3 2 1

For my family

whose love does my heart good
even more than exercise

ACKNOWLEDGMENTS

Though writing a book can be a solitary voyage, I was fortunate to have a number of fellow travelers along the way whose help and support were indispensible.

Brad Kolowich, Jr., my co-author, brought not only his considerable expertise to the book, but also his infectious enthusiasm. His upbeat personality and can-do attitude, which have contributed to his tremendous success as a personal trainer, have also made him an outstanding partner for this project.

I am equally grateful to Ellen Kadin, my wonderful editor at AMACOM, who served as chief guide and cheerleader throughout the process. The talent and hard work of Ellen and her colleagues, along with that of fitness photographer Zach Hawkins, brought to life what had been a long-simmering idea in my head.

Thanks are also due to the individuals who were kind enough to share their inspirational fitness journeys, and to my good friend and longtime colleague Leigh Seaman, who gathered and wrote their stories.

My workout buddy Trevor Rosenthal lent both brains and brawn to the effort, serving as a sounding board as I pondered various aspects of the book, and as an adept exercise tester. I also appreciate the input of my friends Erin Robboy and Josh Norcross, who patiently listened to me talk about the book (or pretended to listen) on our weekly hikes. My mother, Scottie, went well beyond her maternal duties by poring over multiple drafts and offering her unvarnished opinions.

My friend and colleague Loren Goldfarb, on whose wise counsel I rely regularly, provided feedback that, as always, was invaluable. The same goes for my close friend Edward Felsenthal, whose editorial guidance unquestionably made this a better book.

My own fitness journey—and therefore this book—would not have been possible without my first personal trainer, Kevin Kusinski, who is among the best teachers I've ever had. Kevin always kept me laughing during my workouts and wanting to come back for more. I'm also deeply indebted to my friend and current trainer, Chris George, who is one of the most talented fitness professionals in the business. Pushing me beyond what I thought were my limits, Chris has transformed not only my body but also how I feel about it. It's my hope that *Fitter Faster* can help do the same for you.

CONTENTS

Introduction

From first grade on, it was the thing about school I hated most: Not math tests. Not mind-numbing assemblies. Not even the inedible lunches.

It was gym class.

At the all-boys elementary school that I attended, athletic prowess was considered just as important as academic achievement. Consequently, everyone was required to attend daily PE classes, which always began by our lining up and performing calisthenics like jumping jacks, sit-ups, leg lifts, burpees, and crab push-ups. As a chubby kid who didn't especially like sports or sweating, I detested all the exercises. But one I found especially odious was something dubbed "Chinese torture" by the coaches. This involved lying on our stomachs, grabbing our ankles, and rocking back and forth (an exercise that I now know is actually called a "rocking horse").

Leaning back in his chair, the head coach would bark out orders like a drill sergeant as he puffed away on a cigarette. After getting his nic fix, he would have us choose teams—I was not exactly a first-round draft pick—and then play some type of seemingly pointless game. Most often it was Cowboys and Indians (aka dodgeball) in which the object—as best I could tell—was to hurl red rubber balls at players on the other team and try to knock the crap out of them. If you got hit, you were "out" and had to go sit on the bleachers. In what you might call an auto-out, I often purposely got hit (or pretended to) within the first 30 seconds so I could escape the melee and maximize my time comfortably seated on the sidelines with my friend Daniel, who had turned me on to this trick.

My aversion to exertion and efforts to avoid it whenever possible lasted through high school. But things began to change when I got to college. There I developed an interest in health and started reading about the benefits of aerobic exercise. I began jogging, initially for just a few minutes at a time, until eventually I was able to go several miles. Over time, my distance and speed increased, and running became a regular part of my life. Eventually I became interested in other types of exercise as well and started going to the gym to lift weights.

Today I hit the running trails or work out virtually every day, doing many of those same calisthenics that I so dreaded as a child. But now I actually enjoy them and can't imagine my life without regular physical activity. At middle age, I am in the best shape of my life and am able to move my body in ways that I never could have imagined doing when I was young.

So, what changed? Well I'm still far from a star athlete and not a fan of dodgeball. But I've developed a very different relationship with physical activity. That's happened because I discovered an activity that worked for me—running—and from there was able to make exercise a regular part of my life.

And that's my goal in this book for you: to help make exercise less daunting and more doable so you can incorporate it more easily into your life.

UNDERSTANDABLE EXCUSES

There are lots of reasons why many of us find it so difficult to exercise. Let's start with perhaps the most common one: too little time.

Consider the official recommendations from the federal government and health authorities. We're supposed to get at least 30 minutes, five days a week, of moderate aerobic activity (meaning things like brisk walking, biking, or doubles tennis). In addition, we're told that we need two or three days a week of strength-training exercises that target all the major muscle groups. Add to that at least two or three days of stretching exercises. Phew! It can be exhausting just imagining how to fit all that in, much less doing it.

A survey by the Centers for Disease Control and Prevention has found that about 80 percent of American adults fail to meet both the aerobic and strength-training guidelines. That's not surprising, given the time required. The shocking part is that 20 percent manage to comply, though I suspect that a good chunk of them are stretching the truth.

Something else that keeps people from hitting the gym is that they don't like gyms. And it's easy to understand why. Working out alongside spandex-clad people with perfectly sculpted bodies can be intimidating, to say the least. And knowing what exercises to do and how to use the equipment, some of which resembles what you might find in a torture chamber, can be overwhelming. Taking classes can be a solution, but dragging yourself to a 6 A.M. boot camp or ending the day with a pedal-till-you-puke spinning class is many people's idea of hell. The fear of looking silly in front of others also keeps people away from gyms, as does the monthly cost of membership.

Then there's the problem that, for many of us, exercise itself is no fun. Or downright unbearable. That feeling is often reinforced by images we see on TV. Shows like *The Biggest Loser* feature overweight people forced to run on treadmills until they drop while being berated by trainers. I don't know about you, but I can think of lots of things that I'd rather do—cleaning animal cages at the zoo or sitting next to a screaming baby on an airplane among them. Infomercials for programs like P90X or Insanity make exercise look so grueling that I get exhausted just watching from my bed.

BARRIER-LOWERING WORKOUTS

This book is about overcoming those barriers—to redefine exercise so that it's less time-consuming and intimidating, and more convenient and enjoyable. To do that, I've teamed up with personal trainer Brad Kolowich Jr., who has years of experience working with both celebrities and ordinary folks of all ages, sizes, and fitness levels.

Brad and I have developed an easy-to-follow workout plan that requires as little as 15 minutes a day. It provides aerobic, muscle-building, and fat-burning benefits that are similar to—and potentially even greater than—what you'd get from regimens two or three times longer. We accomplish this by incorporating high-intensity interval training (HIIT), in which you go hard, then easy, then hard, and so on for a total of 10 or 15 minutes instead of exercising at a constant rate for 30 minutes or longer. In addition, we use circuits for strength training, in which you move relatively quickly from one exercise to the next and thereby cut the length of your workouts. Some of our routines further increase efficiency by providing aerobic and strength benefits at the same time or working multiple muscle groups. Our regimens are designed as accordions so that on days you have extra time and want to exercise longer, you can easily do so.

All our workouts can be done at home or outdoors, which means you won't need to join a gym or worry about scheduling around gym hours or class times. You can exercise at whatever time of day or night is most convenient for you. No fancy or expensive equipment is required—just a set of dumbbells.

In addition, the *Fitter Faster* plan includes two key features to reduce the drudgery of exercise: choice and variety. If running on a treadmill (or running, period) isn't your thing, no worries. Within the structure we've laid out, you'll be able to choose activities you find most enjoyable, whether walking, hiking, biking, dancing, or doing yoga. What's more, the program is customizable, with beginner, intermediate, and advanced plans, so you can select a level that's right for you and challenge yourself with new exercises as you progress. Further, we mix things up with a different routine every day of the week, which will help prevent boredom.

Of course, lowering barriers is meaningless if an exercise plan doesn't produce results. Ours does. Using the workouts in this book with clients of all types, Brad has seen tremendous improvements in their endurance, strength, and body fat.

Evidence-Based Exercise

You don't have to just take our word for the effectiveness of the *Fitter Faster* plan. Its various components, from HIIT to circuit training to plyometrics (or jumping exercises), are backed by solid science. Lots of it. In the book, I explain the scientific basis for our approach, drawing on reams of research about the most effective methods of aerobic exercise, strength training, and stretching. (Should you wish to review any of the research yourself, there's a lengthy list of references at the end of the book.)

For me, the science is paramount. As a longtime health journalist with academic training in public health, I've spent my career digging into the evidence behind various health practices. My interest in the subject of exercise therefore isn't just personal; it's also professional, fueled by my desire and ability to sift through the science and lay out what it shows as clearly and objectively as I can.

That's especially important when it comes to exercise, a field full of fads, half-truths, and false promises. You can find plenty of self-proclaimed fitness experts on websites and in the media who offer opinions or personal experiences masquerading as evidence. When they do cite research, it may be animal studies (which often have little or no relevance to humans) or small, poorly designed studies in people.

Granted, large clinical trials that prove cause and effect can be hard to come by in exercise science, in part because of the difficulty and expense of conducting them. Still, that doesn't mean that we lack sufficient research to know what works. On many fitness-related issues there's a relatively large body of research that, when taken as a whole, yields strong evidence.

Relying on such research, *Fitter Faster* cuts through the hype and misinformation, telling you what's believable and what's not about various aspects of exercise. Working on the book, I've been repeatedly surprised by what the science reveals, and I suspect you'll have the same reaction to much of what I've found, including why taking 10,000 steps a day may be overrated; why stretching could be detrimental; how regularly changing your strength-training regimen can improve your results; why athletic clothing that keeps you dry may be more likely to stink; why taking painkillers before exercise could be counterproductive; and which dietary supplements are—and are not—proven to enhance workouts.

You'll also get science-backed answers to questions that many of us ask. For example, what's the best time of day to work out? Is too much exercise dangerous? Is it okay to exercise with a cold? What's the best type of exercise for burning fat? Are those ab devices on infomercials really effective? Does more sweating mean a more intense workout? Does jogging hurt your knees? What type of protein supplement is best?

By setting the record straight on a range of issues, I hope to reduce the confusion that can lead us to do the wrong things, waste time and money, and throw up our hands in frustration and say "forget it." With the knowledge that you gain from *Fitter Faster*, you'll be smarter about what to do (and what to ignore) and have greater confidence that you're on the right track.

The book is divided into four sections. Part I, "Get Ready," focuses on the benefits of exercise (some of which you likely haven't heard about), secrets to getting and staying motivated, and workout clothing and equipment that you'll need. Part II, "Get Smart," gives you the lowdown on each of the three components of the *Fitter Faster* program: aerobic exercise, strength training, and stretching. Part III, "Get More Out of Exercise," discusses what you should eat to complement your workouts and how to prevent exercise-related pain. And Part IV, "Get Going," lays out our detailed workout plans, with descriptions and photos of each exercise.

ALL ABOARD!

Throughout the book you'll learn about real people, from a woman in Colorado who discovered that nightly walks calmed her mind and helped her sleep, to a man in New Jersey who thought of exercise as a chore but found joy in returning to his childhood passion of playing ice hockey. Though their journeys are very different, they've all arrived at the same destination of enriched lives because of regular physical activity. It's my hope that some of their stories will inspire you to get moving or keep going.

Whether you're looking to start a fitness routine, get back into exercise, or kick up your workouts a notch, *Fitter Faster* can help you achieve your goals. Though our workout plan is designed for people of all ages and fitness levels, you may need to modify or avoid certain parts if you're pregnant, injured or disabled, or if you have a condition such as arthritis or heart disease. Talk to your health-care provider about how to customize the plan in a way that's safe and effective for you.

Whatever your status, if you're thinking that you're too busy, too out of shape, too overweight, too old, too unathletic, too intimidated, or too whatever to be physically active, I'm here to tell you otherwise. If I—the kid whose idea of nirvana was being excused from gym class—can exercise regularly, anyone can. And I can personally attest to what the research shows: that the rewards, both physical and mental, are enormous.

Yes, you can do it, and I'll tell you how. So let's go!

Get Ready

How to Motivate Yourself and
What to Buy

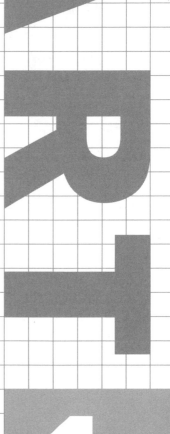

Why Bother?

Before Jillian Michaels, Jack LaLanne, or Jane Fonda, there was Herodicus. While you may not recognize the name, you can credit (or blame) this Greek physician from the fifth century B.C. next time you're urged to exercise for your health.

Herodicus, who had previously been a gym teacher, promoted the then-novel concept that physical activity could keep people healthy. He recommended regimens so strenuous that they might have landed him today on his own version of one of those vomit-inducing DVD workouts.

Many doctors in his day took a dim view of Herodicus and his notions about exercise. But one who listened was his student Hippocrates, who would go on to become one of the most influential physicians in history. Building on Herodicus's teachings, Hippocrates wrote extensively about the health benefits of exercise, observing that "walking is man's best medicine." He also warned about the effects of inactivity: If parts of the body are "unused and left idle," he wrote, "they become liable to disease, defective in growth, and age quickly."

Though many who came after Hippocrates echoed his ideas, it would be more than 2,000 years before British medical researcher Jeremy Morris backed them up with solid scientific evidence. In the 1950s, he showed that double-decker bus drivers in London, who sat for most of their shifts, had more heart attacks and heart-related deaths than the conductors, who spent many of their working hours climbing stairs. (Incidentally, Morris, who acted on his findings and exercised nearly every day, lived to be 99.)

Since Morris's research, there have been thousands of other studies on exercise, and the results are irrefutable: It's good for us in multiple ways. Nothing—no pill, potion, supplement, or diet—even comes close to exercise for being able to do so much for so many people. Or likely ever will.

THE BIG SIX

So what exactly can exercise do for you? Let's start with what I call the Big Six Benefits.

1. Live Longer.

Research shows that elite athletes tend to live longer than the general population. That's certainly good news for Serena Williams, Michael Phelps, and LeBron James. But what about the rest of us?

Well, luckily you don't have to be an athletic superstar for physical activity to extend your life. In fact, the biggest gains in longevity may occur when you go from being a couch potato to taking a short daily walk. When researchers pooled findings from nine studies cumulatively involving more than 120,000 people age 60 and older, they found that those who did moderately intense exercises such as brisk walking or leisurely biking for just 15 minutes a day, five days a week, had a 22 percent lower risk of dying than those who were sedentary.

Similar findings came from a study of more than 330,000 Europeans who were followed for 12 years. Compared to people who didn't exercise at all, those who burned just 100 calories a day through physical activity, which translates to 20 minutes of walking, biking, weeding the garden, or sweeping the floor, had lower mortality rates—even if they were overweight or obese.

Other research suggests that you can further boost longevity by stepping up the pace of your workouts. For example, an Australian study of more than 200,000 people showed that people who devote at least some of their exercise time to vigorous activities such as jogging, fast biking, or singles tennis live longer than those who do the same amount of less vigorous exercise. Another study, which pooled results from 80 studies involving more than a million participants, concluded that those who engaged in vigorous exercise had the lowest risk of death.

Now, before we go any further, I should acknowledge that the concept of a "lower risk of death" sounds odd. Ridiculous, really. As my good friend Edward, who's an editor, likes to point out, we *all* have a 100 percent chance of dying. When researchers use this kind of language, what they mean is that subjects who exercised were less likely to die during the course of the study than those who didn't exercise. Put another way, their risk of *premature* death was lower.

In any case, it's a bit hard to wrap our minds around reductions in mortality risk. An easier way to grasp this is to look at how many years of life we gain by exercising. To that end, researchers in the U.S. pooled results from six studies, which together included more than 650,000 subjects. They found that those who were the most physically active lived an average of 4.5 years longer than people who were inactive.

One shortcoming of all this research is that it relies on subjects reporting their exercise habits on questionnaires. People can have faulty memories, or they may lie. Another problem is that it shows correlations but doesn't prove cause and effect. It's possible, for example, that people who are healthier or genetically programmed to live longer tend to exercise more. But researchers have ways of taking these possibilities into account, and the research as a whole is strong and consistent enough to conclude that regular physical activity can allow us to stick around longer.

Of course, some people may say "no, thanks" to those extra years if they come with a poor quality of life. But research suggests that fitness may lead to a "compression of morbidity"—delaying debilitating conditions until a short time before death so you have more healthy years. As a result, physical activity may add life to your years as well as years to your life.

2. Improve Your Heart Health.

Since Jeremy Morris's groundbreaking research on London bus drivers and their risk of heart disease, countless other studies have reached the same conclusion: People who are physically active have lower rates of heart attacks and strokes than those who are sedentary. They're also less likely to die from these conditions. And we're not talking about just healthy people: Those who have had heart attacks or have cardiovascular disease experience these same benefits.

Exercise appears to work its magic on the cardiovascular system in a number of ways. Studies show that it improves cardiorespiratory fitness, which is a measure of how well the body delivers oxygen to the muscles during exertion, by enhancing the heart's ability to pump blood. Physical activity widens blood vessels and makes them more flexible. It improves cholesterol levels (especially HDL, the good kind) and reduces blood fats called triglycerides along with blood pressure and inflammation, which has been linked to heart attacks and strokes.

What's more, exercise lowers cardiovascular risk through its effect on the body's ability to use insulin, which helps cells absorb glucose from the blood and use it for energy. If cells become resistant to insulin, the result can be elevated blood sugar and, eventually, type 2 diabetes. Both insulin resistance and type 2 diabetes increase the risk of cardiovascular disease. So by improving insulin sensitivity, exercise helps ward off not only type 2 diabetes but also heart disease.

Exercisers who up their intensity appear to benefit even more. A review of studies found that those who engage in intense exercise like jogging have a lower risk of cardiovascular disease than people who do less vigorous activities like walking. Even in people with heart failure, a condition in which the heart is weakened and can't pump enough blood to the body, research shows that more intense exercise results in greater cardiovascular benefits than less intense exercise.

Now, none of this is to say that walking isn't worth the effort; it's unquestionably beneficial. So if that's your thing, by all means keep doing it. But you'll likely be doing the old ticker an even greater favor if you're able and willing to pick up the pace.

3. Cut Your Cancer Risk.

While it's an overstatement to say you can literally walk or run away from cancer, numerous studies suggest that regular exercise may decrease your risk of certain types of cancer. Some of the best evidence is for colon cancer. Pooling results from 52 studies, researchers concluded that people who are physically active have a 24 percent lower risk of the disease than those who are sedentary.

Is too much exercise dangerous?

We've all heard stories of famous athletes who suddenly dropped dead. These tragic events sometimes stoke fears that extremely vigorous exercise may be harmful. In fact, research does suggest that people who engage in extreme endurance sports such as ultramarathon races or professional cycling are more prone to atrial fibrillation, a heart-rhythm abnormality. And extreme exercise may cause temporary, short-term negative effects on the heart, though it's unclear whether these have any lasting impact.

What we do know is that people who die during or after exercise typically have underlying heart problems, and the risk of such deaths is exceedingly low. One study, for example, found that among 11 million participants in marathons and half-marathons, 59 suffered cardiac arrest, 42 of whom died. That translates to a death rate of about 4 in a million. You're more likely to die from crossing the street.

For the vast majority of us, then, any dangers posed by exercise—even vigorous exercise—are dwarfed by the potential benefits. Still, if you've been sedentary and have a condition such as cardiovascular disease, diabetes, or kidney disease, or have symptoms of these conditions, the American College of Sports Medicine recommends seeing your doctor before starting an exercise program. The same goes if you have one of these conditions and are already physically active but want to kick it up to vigorous exercise. And you should stop exercising and get checked out if you develop any symptoms such as chest pain or dizziness.

There's also good evidence linking exercise to a reduced risk of breast cancer. For example, a study of nearly 183,000 postmenopausal women found that those who were the most physically active (at least five days a week) were at lower risk of breast cancer than women who weren't active. The research is less conclusive, though still promising, for other types of cancer including endometrial, lung, liver, bladder, kidney, esophageal, and stomach.

Researchers aren't sure why exercise may ward off cancer, though they theorize that it's due to exercise-induced decreases in inflammation, sex hormones, insulin, or a hormone called IGF-1. Or it could relate to exercise's ability to boost the immune system.

For people who have cancer, exercise has well-established benefits. It reduces fatigue, enhances emotional well-being, and improves quality of life overall. What's more, it may help extend the lives of cancer patients. Research shows that those who were physically active before diagnosis have improved survival rates, as do those who exercise regularly *after* their diagnosis.

4. Boost Your Brain Power.

Second to cancer, Alzheimer's is the most feared disease, according to surveys. And here too exercise may offer protection—or at least delay the disease. A study that followed nearly 20,000 people found that those who were fit in midlife (as determined by treadmill tests) were less likely to develop Alzheimer's disease or other forms of dementia in their 70s and 80s than people who weren't fit.

Many other studies have shown that people who exercise regularly—whether in middle age or later in life—have a lower risk of dementia than those who are sedentary. Physical activity is also associated with a reduced risk of mild cognitive impairment, which involves problems with memory and thinking that are less serious than those seen in dementia but more pronounced than normal age-related memory decline.

While these studies, as a whole, make a compelling case that exercise can benefit our brains, they show only associations. We have more conclusive evidence from randomized trials, which are capable of proving cause and effect. For example, studies involving patients with dementia have found that subjects randomly assigned to supervised exercise programs show improvements on tests of memory and thinking, which generally do not occur in the control (i.e., non-exercising) groups.

Likewise, there's proof from randomized studies that exercise is good for the brains of healthy people. Research in children and young adults shows that a single bout of exercise can improve short-term memory. And in studies of middle-aged and older sedentary adults without dementia, scores on tests of memory, attention, processing speed, and executive function (the ability to plan and make decisions) have improved among subjects assigned to exercise programs.

Further evidence comes from studies in which researchers have studied people's brains using MRI. In a randomized trial of 120 older adults, for example, exercise training increased the size of the hippocampus, a part of the brain involved in memory that typically shrinks as we age. Exercise has also been shown to increase volume in other regions of the brain, including the prefrontal cortex, which regulates executive function and is especially susceptible to age-related shrinkage.

The jury is still out on why, exactly, exercise helps with brain function. One possibility involves a protein called BDNF, which protects nerve cells in the brain, promotes the growth of new ones, and enhances the ability of nerve cells to communicate with one another. Animal and human studies show that exercise increases levels of BDNF.

Another possible explanation is that exercise protects small blood vessels in the brain and improves blood flow there, which helps keep our minds sharp. Put another way, what's good for cardiovascular health may also be good for brain health.

Whatever the reason or reasons for the brain-boosting effects of exercise, studies suggest it needs to be moderately intense or vigorous to do the trick. And a combination of aerobic exercise and strength training appears to be more beneficial than either alone.

5. Improve Your Mood.

We've all heard of runner's high, that sense of euphoria that some people get from vigorous exercise. While most of us will never experience it (and may instead associate exercise with just the opposite), research shows that physical activity can give you a milder version of this feeling in the form of an improved mood. And you don't have to run a marathon or do an Ironman triathlon to see this benefit.

More than two dozen studies have found that people who exercise regularly have a lower risk of developing depression. One of these studies, which followed 11,000 people over three decades, found that the more frequently they worked out, the fewer symptoms of depression they had.

In addition, a review of 35 randomized trials concluded that exercise can reduce symptoms in people who have depression—perhaps as effectively as medication or therapy in some cases. Other studies show that physical activity can help alleviate anxiety.

Researchers have several theories as to why exercise helps fight depression and anxiety. One possibility is that it increases levels of mood-boosting brain chemicals such as endorphins (which act like morphine) and endocannabinoids (which act like marijuana). Exercise may also help by providing social interaction, boosting self-confidence, or distracting us from things that stress us.

Some of these factors may also explain why people without depression or anxiety also benefit psychologically from exercise. Studies show it can give you an enhanced sense of well-being and greater energy that last for several hours. That's certainly true for me: After a workout I feel more relaxed and am better able to handle life's everyday annoyances. I also tend to be more productive.

What's more, physical activity can make you more creative. For example, one study found that college students performed better on tests of creativity while they were walking (either on a treadmill or outside) than when seated. The creativity boost appeared to continue after the walks ended. As the researchers put it, exercise "opens up the free flow of ideas."

6. Fend Off Feebleness.

It's an unhappy fact, but our bone density peaks around the ripe old age of 30. In the decades that follow, we gradually lose bone, along with muscle strength, and the risk of joint problems rises. Eventually this musculoskeletal decline can lead to pain, weakness, and disability that we typically associate with advancing age. But regular exercise can slow

TAMMI
AGE 40
BOULDER, COLORADO

Sleep just would not come for Tammi. It wasn't hard to understand why. Her mother's recent death and the fragile state of her marriage created stress that kept her mind buzzing long after the lights went out. One night around 4 A.M., Tammi pulled sweats on over her pajamas and went for a walk on the quiet streets of her sleeping neighborhood. The walk helped, and she slept well once back in her bed. She walked the next night and the night after that. After about a week, she realized that the walks were helping to calm her racing mind.

Soon, Tammi was falling asleep at a regular hour and didn't need the nighttime strolls, so she set her alarm for dawn and walked before work. "The calm, meditative focus was a first for me," Tammi says. "I had been living my life with such intensity, not realizing the damage I was doing to myself physically, emotionally, and spiritually." The steps Tammi took on her walks led to steps designed to improve her life: changing jobs, ending an unhealthy marriage, and focusing more on wellness.

Those changes helped her deal with the shocking news two years later that she had an aggressive form of breast cancer. The treatments were physically grueling, but Tammi returned to her walks as soon as she could. Eventually she moved her family to a community where she and her daughters could walk virtually everywhere they needed to go. Now more than five years cancer-free and facing a healthy future, Tammi is hiking mountains. "Movement literally saved my life," Tammi says. "Twice."

17

or halt this deterioration, allowing older bodies to function like much younger ones.

So-called weight-bearing exercises, which force you to work against gravity, are best for your bones. These include running, hiking, brisk walking, jumping rope, climbing stairs, playing tennis, and lifting weights—but not swimming or biking (which are beneficial in other ways, though). A review of 43 randomized studies involving postmenopausal women found that subjects assigned to do such exercises experienced less bone loss in the spine and hip than those who didn't exercise. Other studies show the same for men. By slowing or stopping bone loss, exercise can reduce the risk of osteoporosis and fractures.

In addition, exercise increases muscle mass and strength. A review of more than 120 randomized studies concluded that older people who engaged in strength training had an improved ability to walk, climb steps, and stand up from a chair. Increased strength may also mean a lower risk of falls—an especially important benefit, given that they can lead to broken hips, loss of independence, and death in older people.

Other research suggests that physical activity—especially vigorous activities—may reduce the risk of osteoarthritis (the most common form of arthritis) by strengthening cartilage, which cushions joints. Exercise has also been shown to improve physical function and decrease joint pain in people who have that condition.

Some of the best evidence that exercise can serve as a fountain of youth comes from elite older athletes who participate in competitions like marathons, triathlons, or track meets. Research shows that they don't have the deterioration of bones, muscles, and joints seen in others their age, nor do they experience the same physical limitations. What this suggests is that the age-related breakdown in our bodies may have more to do with how much we move them than how many birthdays we've had.

Obviously, very few of us participate in Ironman races or sprinting contests (or even aspire to), but you don't have to be an elite athlete—or any kind of athlete—to experience the age-defying effects of exercise. Even frail nursing-home residents in their 80s and 90s have been shown to gain muscle strength from exercising. The key is to incorporate different kinds of exercise and, of course, to keep doing them regularly.

THE SURPRISING SEVEN

In addition to extending life and reducing the risk of deadly or debilitating conditions, regular exercise can enhance the quality of your life, sometimes in ways you might not expect. Here are seven benefits that may surprise you.

1. Have Better Sex.

In men, regular exercise appears to be a natural Viagra: It's associated with a lower risk of erectile problems. In one study, sedentary middle-aged men assigned to participate in a vigorous exercise program for nine months reported more frequent sexual activity, improved sexual function, and greater satisfaction. Those whose fitness levels increased the most saw the biggest improvements in their sex lives.

Research in women has found that those who are physically active report greater sexual desire, arousal, and satisfaction than women who are sedentary. In one unusual experiment, young women who did intense cycling for 20 minutes and watched an X-rated film showed greater physiological sexual arousal (as measured by a device that assesses vaginal blood flow) than subjects who did not exercise before seeing the film.

Increased blood flow helps explain why exercise leads to better sexual function in men as well. An enhanced self-image from exercise may play a role too. Men and women who exercise may be more likely to feel sexually desirable, which can lead to better sex. So can the greater strength, flexibility, and stamina that result from exercise.

In addition, physical activity—especially strength training—can increase levels of testosterone, which may boost sex drive in men and women. It's worth noting that overtraining can have the opposite effect by lowering testosterone levels. While this is a potential concern for elite athletes or others who push themselves to the max without adequate recovery, it's not something that most of us need to worry about.

Does sex before physical activity impair athletic performance?

In ancient times, abstinence from sex was considered essential for success in sports. Since then, many coaches have discouraged pre-competition sex, believing that it reduces aggression and strength. As Rocky Balboa's trainer put it in the movie *Rocky*, "women weaken legs."

A review of studies, however, found little support for the belief. One of them, which involved former male athletes, measured grip strength the morning after they'd had sex with their wives and then repeated the test after the men had abstained for at least six days. There were no differences in test results. Similarly, another study in male athletes found that sexual activity didn't affect performance on a cycle stress test. However, subjects who'd had sex two hours before the test had higher heart rates during post-exercise recovery.

Overall, the research suggests that sex before physical activity doesn't have negative effects as long as there's a lag of at least two hours and the sexual activity doesn't also involve alcohol, drugs, or sleep loss. In fact, it's possible that sex may even enhance athletic performance by helping people relax.

But much remains unknown, including whether women are affected differently than men. It's likely that the impact of sex on physical activity varies from person to person. As a result, if you're wondering how pre-game sex affects your golf score or your 5K race time, you'll need to do your own experiment and see for yourself.

2. Sleep More Soundly.

The headline of a survey by the National Sleep Foundation said it best: "Exercise is good for sleep." In the poll of 1,000 people, those who exercised the most vigorously reported the best sleep quality overall. And they were less likely than non-exercisers to say that in the past two weeks they had experienced problems such as trouble falling asleep or waking up during the night.

These findings are supported by a review of 66 studies on exercise and sleep. It concluded that regular exercise is comparable to sleep medication or behavioral therapy in improving the ability to fall asleep, as well as sleep duration and quality. Researchers aren't sure why, but they suspect physical activity may help by affecting body temperature, metabolic rate, heart rate, or anxiety levels, among other things.

Because exercise also revs up your body, conventional wisdom has it that exercising in the evening can interfere with sleep. But overall, research has failed to support this assertion. For example, a small study of young adults found that doing vigorous aerobic exercise two hours before bedtime did not impair sleep quality. Likewise, a study in elderly people showed that low-impact aerobic workouts done between 7:00 and 8:30 in the evening were just as effective as morning workouts at improving self-reported sleep quality.

Of course, everyone is different, so it's possible that nighttime exercise may make it harder for you to sleep. But the only way to know for sure is to try. So, if like me, you find that evenings are the most convenient time to lace up your sneakers, don't be scared off by fears of insomnia. You may be pleasantly surprised at what a little pre-bedtime sweat can do for your sleep.

3. Catch Fewer Colds.

You may have heard fitness buffs claim that they never get sick. While this may seem like baseless—not to mention annoying—boasting, there is scientific truth to it. Numerous studies have linked regular exercise to a lower risk of colds. For example, a study that followed 1,000 adults for three months found that those who did aerobic exercise at least five days a week were about half as likely to develop colds as those who didn't exercise. And when exercisers did catch colds, they had fewer and less severe symptoms than their couch-potato peers.

These studies, which show associations but not cause and effect, are corroborated by randomized trials on exercise and colds. In one such experiment involving sedentary postmenopausal women, participants were assigned to either moderately intense exercise (such as brisk walking) five days a week or once-a-week stretching. By the final three months of the 12-month study, those doing regular exercise reported having substantially fewer colds than the stretchers.

Research in animals and humans suggests that exercise chases away colds by boosting the immune system. At the same time, very intense activities may *suppress* immunity by increasing levels of the stress hormones cortisol and adrenaline. That perhaps explains why, in one study, runners who participated in a Los Angeles marathon were nearly six times more likely to get sick in the week after the race than runners who did not participate.

While this is a potential issue for elite athletes or people who do marathons or triathlons, the level of activity among most exercisers—even if it's vigorous—is far more likely to keep colds at bay than bring them on.

4. Avoid Back Pain.

Like the common cold, low back pain afflicts most people at some point in their lives. It's the leading cause of job-related disability and can interfere with everyday activities. Though claims abound about various measures that supposedly can prevent it, the only one that's actually been shown to work is regular exercise.

In a review of more than 20 studies that examined various back-pain prevention techniques, exercise was the clear winner over measures such as back belts and shoe insoles. It reduced the odds of not only experiencing back pain but also missing work due to the condition.

The type of exercise didn't appear to matter. Activities focused on aerobic conditioning, strength, balance, and flexibility all seemed to be effective. Exercises that strengthen core muscles—which include those in the abdomen, back, and hips—help by supporting the spine. General exercise regimens can have the same effect by increasing muscle

Is it okay to exercise with a cold?

For some people, exercise may be the last thing they want to do when they're sniffling and sneezing with a cold. But for others, that's not enough to keep them on the couch, and science suggests that exercise is probably fine as long as symptoms are above the neck—meaning a runny nose, sore throat, or head congestion. In one study, researchers caused subjects to develop such symptoms by spraying a cold virus into their noses. (Finding volunteers for this study likely wasn't easy!) Some participants were then randomly assigned to exercise, while the others served as controls. Physical activity appeared to have no negative effects: The exercisers' colds weren't any longer or more severe than those of the non-exercisers. If anything, the exercisers fared a bit better.

The upshot is that you likely won't do yourself harm and may even feel better if you exercise with a garden-variety cold. But if you have more serious symptoms such as fever, extreme fatigue, swollen glands, or a chest cough, you should lay off exercise until you recover.

Regardless of your symptoms, it's worth heeding the rule of my germophobic trainer Kevin Kusinski: Never go to the gym sick. The fact that fitness facilities typically have lots of people in close contact touching the same equipment, not to mention dripping sweat and sometimes spewing saliva onto it, makes gyms hotbeds of germ transmission. The standard precautions of wiping down equipment after using it and covering your nose and mouth (which isn't exactly doable when you sneeze while, say, holding two dumbbells aloft) often aren't adequate to prevent the spread of germs in a gym. So if you want to exercise when you have a cold, go for it, but keep your germs to yourself by doing your workout at home or outdoors. Your fellow gymgoers will thank you.

strength and endurance as well as preventing weight gain, which puts added stress on the back. In addition, physical activity can help by alleviating anxiety and depression, which in some cases may contribute to back pain.

Exercise can head off back pain in the first place, or reduce the chances of its recurring if you've had the condition before. But for that to happen, you need to keep exercising after the pain goes away. Once you stop, so do the protective benefits.

5. Preserve Your Eyesight.

When you hear about a connection between exercise and eyesight, maybe you picture those eye-exercise programs that promise to sharpen your vision. But that's not what we're talking about. Instead of moving your eyes, the idea is to move your feet.

Research shows that people who are physically active have a lower risk of cataracts. For example, a study of nearly 50,000 runners and walkers found that those who exercised most vigorously were 42 percent less likely to develop cataracts than those who exercised least vigorously. Exercisers who fell in the middle in terms of intensity were also at reduced risk, though to a lesser degree.

The same researcher found a similar benefit regarding age-related macular degeneration (AMD), a leading cause of vision loss, in a study of nearly 42,000 runners. The more that people ran, the more their risk of AMD declined. A different study, which followed roughly 4,000 people for 15 years, showed that participants who were physically active were less likely to develop AMD than those who weren't active.

Scientists aren't sure why exercise protects against cataracts and AMD. One possibility is that it reduces inflammation, which is associated with both conditions. Cataracts and AMD have also been linked to risk factors for cardiovascular disease, including elevated blood sugar and triglycerides, which regular exercise can lower. Further, some research suggests that people who are overweight or obese are more prone to cataracts and AMD, so physical activity may help by preventing weight gain.

6. Protect Your Hearing.

You heard it here first: Exercise may be good for your hearing. A study of more than 68,000 female nurses who were followed for 20 years found that walking at least two hours a week was associated with a lower risk of hearing loss. Other research has linked higher fitness levels with better hearing.

Exercise may protect against hearing loss by improving blood flow to the cochlea, the snail-shaped structure in the inner ear that converts sound waves into nerve signals that are sent to the brain. What's more, it may prevent the loss of neurotransmitters, which carry those signals between nerve cells. Exercise may also help by reducing the risk of diabetes and cardiovascular disease, both of which are linked to hearing loss.

Of course, blasting music into your ears while you exercise could have the opposite effect and damage your hearing. One study found that people cranked up the volume on their listening devices to dangerously high levels when exposed to noise levels typically found in a fitness facility. The music was even louder when the participants exercised, perhaps to provide motivation. (For more on how music can motivate you, see page 36.)

The longer you listen, the lower the volume needs to be to protect your hearing. For a 60-minute workout, for example, experts recommend keeping the sound at 60 percent or less of the maximum volume level. Noise-canceling headphones are a good option because they reduce the need to turn up your music as much. But don't use them while exercising on a busy road. By being unaware of approaching traffic, you could be subjecting yourself to a risk far more serious than loud music.

7. Pee Less & Poop More.

Okay, I admit it's a bit gross, but this list wouldn't be complete without mentioning the effects of exercise on our ability to go to the bathroom.

The place to start, naturally, is number 1. While high-impact activities like jumping or running can cause women to leak urine, research shows that moderate exercise can decrease the risk. For example, a study of middle-aged female nurses found that those who were physically active had lower rates of urinary incontinence than women who were inactive. A study of older nurses by the same team of researchers yielded similar findings.

A urinary problem familiar to many middle-aged and older men is nocturia, which is the need to get up more than once a night to pee. Often the cause is an enlarged prostate—a condition known as benign prostatic hyperplasia or BPH. Exercise can help prevent nocturia or reduce its severity. In a large study of men with BPH, for example, those who were physically active for an hour or more per week were less likely to report nocturia than those who were sedentary. Likewise, a study of sedentary older men found that after eight weeks of daily walking, they urinated less frequently during the night.

Another common bathroom-related problem for both men and women is constipation, which exercise can help improve as well. In a study of 62,000 women, those who reported daily physical activity were almost half as likely to experience constipation as women who exercised less than once a week. A randomized trial involving inactive, middle-aged men and women with chronic constipation found that those assigned to a 12-week exercise program were able to poop more easily.

Exercise helps by decreasing transit time. That's how long it takes food to move through the digestive tract—not, as it sounds, the amount of time it takes to get to work. Alas, a shorter commute is one benefit that exercise may not have—unless, of course, biking to work is faster for you than driving in heavy traffic.

WAIT . . . WHAT ABOUT WEIGHT?

At this point you may be wondering why I didn't list weight loss among the benefits of exercise. After all, it's the main reason that many of us work out. Certainly TV shows like *The Biggest Loser*, where contestants are subjected to intense exercise regimens and tormentor-trainers, give the impression that exercise is just as crucial as dieting for shedding pounds, if not more so. But the truth is that despite all its health benefits, exercise may have limited effects when it comes to weight loss.

Let's start with how physical activity is most likely to help: by preventing weight gain. Research shows that people who exercise regularly tend to put on less weight. For example, a study that followed participants for 20 years found that the most active men gained six fewer pounds, on average, than their inactive peers as they transitioned from young adulthood into middle age. Active women saw an even greater benefit, gaining an average of 13 fewer pounds than more sedentary women. The researchers controlled for other factors that might explain the findings, including calories consumed.

Similarly, there's evidence that exercise can help you avoid regaining lost weight. The National Weight Control Registry, which studies people who have lost at least 30 pounds and kept it off long-term, reports that many of them exercise an hour or more a day. Research involving overweight and obese women had a similar finding: Those who were most successful at maintaining weight loss after 24 months reported doing relatively vigorous exercise for nearly an hour a day on average. Participants who did less exercise tended to be less successful at keeping the weight off.

When it comes to *losing* weight, however, the research as a whole shows that exercise, whether alone or combined with diet, typically has little effect. So if exercise burns calories, as we're repeatedly reminded, how can this be?

For starters, it takes a lot of exercise—more than most people are willing or able to do—to make much of a dent in our weight or body shape. To lose a pound of fat, you need to burn 3,500 more calories than you take in. Thirty minutes of brisk walking by someone weighing 150 pounds burns only about 140 calories. Add to that the fact that simply sitting in a chair can burn 50, so the net benefit from walking is less than 100 calories. Step it up to running for 30 minutes and you burn around 300 calories net. That's roughly the equivalent of one Starbucks blueberry muffin.

While exercise may make a small contribution, forgoing muffins and other foods is the easier path to weight loss. Achieving it with exercise alone would require roughly five days of 60-minute intense aerobic workouts such as fast-paced cycling, running, or jumping rope. And that's for losing one pound a week.

From there the math becomes more complicated and stacked even more against us. As you lose weight, your metabolism slows and you actually burn fewer calories from the same activities. Though it seems like a cruel joke, it's one of the body's mechanisms for keeping us from

Can sitting cancel out the benefits of exercise?

You've probably heard the trendy phrase that "sitting is the new smoking." While it's an exaggeration to equate the two behaviors—nothing comes close to smoking in its many ruinous and deadly effects on the body—research does show that prolonged sitting may be harmful, even if you exercise regularly.

Pooling results from more than 40 studies, researchers concluded that the more time people spend on their duffs—whether at a desk, on the couch, or in the car—the greater their risk of premature death, cardiovascular disease, cancer, and especially type 2 diabetes. Regular exercise, particularly higher levels of physical activity, appears to blunt these harmful effects somewhat but may not eliminate them entirely.

The damage from prolonged sitting is thought to be due to reduced muscle activity—especially in the large muscles of the legs and back—which can decrease the body's ability to regulate blood sugar and remove harmful blood fats.

To reduce sitting time:
- At work, stand up for a few minutes every half hour, perhaps during phone calls, coffee breaks, or meetings.
- If possible, use a desk that lets you work both standing and seated. Or try one attached to a treadmill that allows you to slowly walk while you work.
- At home, get up regularly from your computer. Try standing and doing chores while watching TV.

Incorporating short bursts of standing and movement like this will keep you from becoming an "active couch potato"—someone who exercises and then remains largely sedentary the rest of the time. By thinking of fitness as something that entails what you do the entire day—not just the relatively few minutes spent sweating—you'll be able to fully reap the rewards of your workouts.

wasting away. To circumvent this and continue losing weight through exercise, you likely need to keep ratcheting up the amount or intensity.

Another reason exercise may not peel away the pounds is that it can prompt you to eat more. Though the evidence is mixed, research finds that physical activity may make us hungrier. (It also can have the opposite effect and suppress appetite.) Even if exercise doesn't affect appetite, it may leave some people feeling entitled to consume more calories because of their hard work at the gym—an attitude reflected in the "I exercise so I can eat" mantra that I often hear people repeat. When I gently inform them how much they need to exert themselves to compensate for those glazed doughnuts at work or extra slices of pizza at dinner, their reactions often include shock, disappointment, denial, or some combination of the three.

Lest I leave you feeling similarly disillusioned, I hasten to emphasize that even if physical activity doesn't make you skinnier, it will make you healthier. Research shows that people who are overweight and fit live longer than those who are slim and unfit. And regular exercise can help reduce many of the health risks associated with being overweight. What's more, strength training can improve your appearance by increasing muscle mass.

Too often, people start an exercise program with unrealistic expectations about what it can do for their weight. When the pounds don't melt away, they become discouraged and give up. Don't let that happen to you. Though the *Fitter Faster* workouts may indeed be more effective than conventional exercise at burning fat, that shouldn't be your only motive for exercising. There are plenty of other compelling reasons to get moving and keep going.

Avoid Off-Ramps

"I didn't make it to the gym today," goes a popular joke. "That makes five years in a row." Indeed, how to consistently turn intention into action is something that most of us struggle with when it comes to physical activity. You might call it the holy grail of exercise. Despite what Nike tells us, "just do it" doesn't cut it. Nor, for most people, does sheer willpower. We face an array of potential obstacles—including jobs, family responsibilities, dislike of exercise, lack of energy, or simple inertia—that often keep us from getting started or knock us off track once we do start. But there are ways to avoid these exercise off-ramps. In this chapter I'll describe some relatively simple measures that can increase your odds of success by reframing the way you think about exercise and making it more convenient, attainable, and enjoyable.

SEEK INSTANT GRATIFICATION

As important as the long-term health benefits of exercise are, simply being aware of them isn't enough to motivate most people. If it were, we'd all be breaking a sweat every day. Instead, research suggests you should focus on the more immediate benefits.

A study of middle-aged women found that subjects whose main goal was to lose weight, live longer, or be healthier actually exercised *less* than those with "quality of life" goals such as more energy or less stress. Put another way, they were more likely to work out if they viewed exercise as a way to enhance their daily lives now rather than something that might pay off in the distant future.

This certainly makes sense, given human nature. We tend to be more motivated by immediate results than ones that seem far off. If I think exercise will help me cope better today with a stressful job or screaming kids, that's more likely to get me to the gym than the notion that exercise will help me avoid a heart attack in 20 years.

The key is identifying what the short-term payoff of exercise is for you. Is it sounder sleep? A better mood? Clearer thinking? Improved digestion? Less pain? More patience? Better sex? A sense of accomplishment? Such benefits may not be instantly evident if you're new to exercise, so determining which ones apply to you can take a little time. But once you figure it out, keep those rewards in mind—or, better yet, post them on your refrigerator, bathroom mirror, or anywhere else you can readily see them—so they provide a nudge, especially when you feel your willpower flagging.

MAKE A WINNING GOAL

Setting specific, measurable goals is also key to staying motivated. Determine what you'd like to accomplish and when you plan to do it. A vague wish such as "I want to walk more" isn't enough. Instead, your goal should be something precise like "I will be walking twice as far six weeks from now." Write it down where you can see it and when you achieve one goal, set another.

While your goal should be challenging—one that's too easy probably won't be very motivating—it shouldn't be unrealistic. For example, if you've never run before, it's not reasonable to expect to run a marathon in a month. Nor, as discussed in chapter 2, is it realistic to think that walking for 30 minutes a day will give you a beach body. Setting goals such as these can lead to discouragement and cause you to give up when you fail to achieve them.

If you set a goal and then realize that it's too hard, modify it. Likewise, if it turns out to be too easy, make it more challenging. Setting the right goals for yourself will likely involve some trial and error, especially at the beginning of an exercise program.

Be sure to keep track of your progress toward your goal. For some people, wearable fitness trackers or smartphone apps can be useful by providing hard data and encouragement. (For more on trackers, see pages 57–59.) But don't feel compelled to go high-tech if that's not your thing. Keeping a journal of your activity—whether on your computer or with pen and paper—is perfectly fine. What's important is to record your activity, in whatever way works for you, so you can see how well you're doing.

HAVE A GAME PLAN

Getting derailed by daily events happens to all of us. Sometimes missing a workout is unavoidable because of an emergency or other unexpected event. But in most cases, inadequate time management is to blame. The solution is to plan ahead and make physical activity a priority.

Think of exercise as an important appointment. Schedule it on your calendar, just as you would any other activity such as your child's soccer game or dinner with friends. If you plan to exercise away from home, be prepared by packing a bag with what you'll need—whether clothing, sneakers, sunglasses, a water bottle, towel, or exercise mat—and setting it by the door the night before. Keeping a packed bag of "emergency" fitness clothing and accessories in your car can be useful as well, in case you forget something or have an unplanned opportunity to work out.

Just as your goals should be realistic, so should your planning. For example, if you tend to be too tired or busy with family duties at the end of the day, don't schedule a workout then; find another time that's better suited to you. Likewise, if you plan to exercise at a park or a gym, choose one that's nearby. The farther out of your way you have to go to work out, the more likely you are to blow it off.

Similarly, don't let bad weather be an excuse for skipping your workout. Check the forecast ahead of time if you intend to exercise outdoors. If it's going to be too hot, too cold, too rainy, or too icy to exercise, plan to do so at home or another indoor location. If you're going to be traveling, check the weather at your destination and pack accordingly. If possible, stay somewhere that has a fitness facility or an outdoor exercise area nearby.

It's also important to have a backup plan. Try to identify what might thwart your exercise plans on a given day—a meeting that could run long, for example—and figure out what you can do in response, such as exercising later in the evening or moving your routine to the next day. However, be careful about pushing your workouts to the weekend, when you may have even more distractions that keep you from exercising.

At this point you may be thinking that this all sounds great in theory—but in reality, you're just too busy. If so, track for several days how you're spending your time. How much of it is devoted to Facebook or Twitter? Texting? Surfing the Internet? Checking e-mails? Watching TV shows? Most of us spend more time on such things than we realize or are willing to admit. With the *Fitter Faster* program, all you need for a good workout is 15 minutes. If you can cut that out of your texting, tweeting, and TV watching, you'll have enough time for fitness.

ENJOY YOURSELF

"Fun" may not be the first word that comes to mind when you think about exercise. But there are ways you can make exercise more enjoyable, which will increase your odds of sticking with it.

For starters, try to find activities that you like—or at least don't mind. On certain days, the *Fitter Faster* program lets you choose whatever activity you prefer, whether it's taking a walk, going for a hike, riding a bike, swimming laps, going dancing, or playing tennis. In short, you should choose whatever floats your boat, and try to mix it up so you don't get bored.

Whenever possible, exercise outdoors. Even if your surroundings don't include tranquil lakes or scenic vistas, the sights and sounds you experience outside can enhance your workout. Indeed, studies have found that people report greater enjoyment from outdoor activities than indoor ones. They're also more likely to do outdoor activities again.

What's the best time of day to exercise?

Some fitness gurus recommend working out first thing in the morning because that's when you're least likely to have scheduling conflicts and therefore more likely to exercise regularly. Plus early exercisers often say that a morning routine leaves them feeling more energized and productive during the day.

But if, like me, you are not a morning person and shudder at the thought of getting out of bed for a 6 A.M. workout, I have good news: We perform best at exercise (especially high-intensity exercise) in the late afternoon. That's when perceived exertion (meaning how hard you feel that your body is working) tends to be lowest. Scientists attribute this effect to our circadian rhythm, the body's 24-hour clock, which causes body temperature to rise slightly throughout the day and peak in late afternoon.

Of course, none of this means that you're doomed to a subpar workout if you exercise in the morning. By doing so consistently, you can eliminate the morning performance gap, according to research, which shows that athletes who train in the morning improve their performance to levels seen in the afternoon. That's worth keeping in mind if you're planning to run, say, a 5K with a 7 A.M. start time: Your performance will be best if you train at that hour.

All in all, the best time to work out is whenever you can do so. If you exercise at different times of the day, be sure to note the hour as you're tracking your progress. That way, you'll know when your body clock may be to blame for a less-than-optimal workout.

AVOID OFF-RAMPS

Other research shows that people's expected enjoyment of exercise is disproportionately influenced by how they view the *beginning* of the workout—a phenomenon that researchers call "forecasting myopia." If your routine includes different exercises and you start with one that you dread, you're more likely to see exercise as unpleasant. If, on the other hand, you begin with your favorite exercise and save your least favorite for last, research suggests you may view exercise as more enjoyable. Keep this in mind when you're doing the *Fitter Faster* strength training and plyometric workouts in chapter 10. If you prefer some exercises over others, feel free to change the order and start with the one you like most.

Whether you're doing multiple activities or just one, looking beyond the initial stage of your workout (which is typically the most unpleasant part) and focusing on the experience as a whole can make it seem more appealing.

Turning exercise into a game can also make it more enjoyable. A growing number of fitness apps immerse users in adventures such as running from zombies, fighting aliens, escaping from Alcatraz, or saving the world. A randomized study of two such apps, The Walk and Zombies, Run!, found that participants who used them reported greater motivation to exercise regularly. And they were more likely to keep exercising during the 12-week study than participants who didn't use the apps.

Like fitness-game apps, other forms of entertainment such as books on tape, podcasts, movies, or TV shows can reduce boredom while you work out and provide a distraction from any discomfort you're feeling. Saving certain entertainment—a series on Netflix you've been wanting to watch, for example—for only when you're exercising can be especially motivating. That way, you'll have something to look forward to and associate your workout with a treat that you don't otherwise get. Just make sure you don't get so engrossed that you neglect proper form or safety.

Perhaps the most potent form of entertainment during exercise is music. A large body of research shows music can enhance the enjoyment of even very strenuous exercise and increase the likelihood of sticking with a fitness program. These effects are due in part to music's ability to decrease how hard we think we're working. Listening to music has been found to boost endurance and performance—a fact not lost on elite athletes who rely on music to help them train. Costas Kara-

EMILY

AGE 76

KNOXVILLE, TENNESSEE

Before she retired, Emily characterized herself as active enough to stay healthy. Her job as a social worker kept her sitting in a chair for long stretches on most days. She exercised occasionally but had no regular fitness routine. It wasn't until Emily became a grandmother that she realized "active enough" didn't cut it when it came to getting on the floor to play with toddlers.

So Emily decided to get more physical activity. As part of her new fitness regimen, she began walking a couple of miles through her neighborhood. As her strength and endurance increased, so did her distance. Emily soon found that she preferred the trails of the nearby national park, where she enjoyed a new appreciation for the beauty of all four seasons.

After ascending to an elevation of over 6,500 feet at age 70, she was inspired to share the physical, mental, and spiritual benefits that she got while hiking. She organized friends to hike with her and soon created a formal hiking group through her church.

Emily now leads twice-monthly hikes for anyone of any age who wants to join her. "I'm not a fitness guru," says Emily, whose now-teenage grandsons often accompany her hiking. "In fact, I think people who might be scared of the words 'hike' or 'mountain' are less intimidated when they realize they're being led by a 76-year-old grandmother. My goal is simply to get people to move off the couch and into the outdoors to reap the benefits of fresh air and being active."

georghis, a psychologist at London's Brunel University and a leading expert on the link between music and physical activity, goes so far as to call music a "type of legal performance-enhancing drug."

But not all songs are created equal when it comes to exercise. Research by Karageorghis and others has found that tunes with 125 to 140 beats per minute are optimal during a workout and that songs at the lower end of this range are best suited for higher-intensity exercise. To figure out the tempo of your favorite tunes, check out websites such as songbpm.com or beatsperminuteonline.com.

Loud music can be more motivating, but resist the urge to crank up the volume all the way if you're wearing headphones, since this can damage your hearing. (For more on this, see page 25.) Lyrics also make a difference. Songs whose words and messages you find energizing or inspiring are more likely to keep you moving. Whether that means "Let It Roll" by Flo Rida or "Let It Go" from *Frozen* is your call.

BE SOCIABLE

Working out with a buddy is yet another way to make exercise more enjoyable. Teaming up with a friend or friends to bike, do yoga, or take a hike, for example, turns exercise into a social occasion that can help make the time pass more quickly. The same goes for working out with a group or taking a fitness class—assuming you enjoy the company of the other people in it. And research shows that the camaraderie can up your game. Studies of people who participate in walking groups, for instance, find that they get more exercise than walkers who go it alone.

But greater enjoyment isn't the only reason that working out with others increases motivation. It can also make you more accountable. You're more likely to show up if you know that someone is expecting you and that failing to make it will let them down. Obviously, the right partner is crucial. You don't want your buddy letting *you* down, so he or she needs to be committed to working out. That person should have a similar schedule so you both can exercise at the same time. (Early-bird and evening exercisers aren't a good match, for example.) And you and your partner should have similar fitness goals and be interested in doing similar types of exercise.

Ideally, a workout buddy should also be in somewhat better shape than you are. That's because exercising with someone who's more capable than we are motivates us to try harder than we would alone—a phenomenon known as the Kohler effect. This has been demonstrated in studies, including one involving 58 college-age women who were randomly assigned to ride a stationary bike either by themselves or with a virtual partner who was in a separate lab. The partners, whom subjects "met" via a pre-recorded Skype session, didn't actually exist. The women were told that their partner's bike-riding performance, which they could track with a "live" feed that was actually a recording, was somewhat better than their own.

Women who believed they were riding alongside a partner pedaled, on average, for about 85 percent longer than those who rode alone. In an interesting twist, the researchers told some partnered subjects that they were part of a team whose overall performance was determined by the "weakest link"—the teammate who gave out first. Women led to believe that they were on this team rode the longest—more than twice as long as the solo riders. Clearly, the pressure not to let down the team, combined with the desire to keep up with the competition, motivated these subjects to work especially hard. This boost in motivation happens when others around you are just moderately better than you. If they're far more advanced at an activity, the result can be just the opposite: You may be more likely to get discouraged and quit. That's why if you're, say, just beginning to jog, it's probably not wise to work out with triathletes.

Of course, finding a suitable workout partner or group isn't always possible. And some people simply prefer to go it alone. If you're a solo exerciser, you may still be able to get the motivational benefits of a workout buddy or group via social media. Whether you're sharing with friends or strangers, you can post results, report your progress, compare notes, swap advice, and receive (and give) virtual pats on the back. In a study of people who participated in a web-based walking program, those who were randomly assigned to an online community where they could communicate with other walkers were more likely to stick with the four-month program than those who had no access to the community.

Many fitness social networks allow you to upload data from your fitness tracker and even compete with others if you're so inclined. And unlike your (non-exercising) followers on Facebook or Twitter, fellow

Can motivation to exercise be "contagious"?

Research suggests that health-related behaviors, both good and bad, can spread like viruses. People are more likely to become obese, for example, if they have a friend who becomes obese. Likewise, a smoker's chances of quitting increase if a spouse, sibling, or friend kicks the habit.

The same type of "social contagion," as researchers call it, may apply to exercise. You may be more motivated to work out if you're surrounded by physically active people—even if you never exercise with them. Evidence comes from a study of 3,800 residents of New York City. Those with active friends reported getting more than twice as much weekly exercise as those without active friends. People with active neighbors were also more likely to be active themselves. Though the study shows an association, not cause and effect, the researchers took into account other factors that might have affected the findings, such as education, income, race, ethnicity, and age.

Research also shows that your significant other can influence you to exercise. In one study, researchers asked approximately 3,300 heterosexual married couples in the U.S. about their physical activity and then did so again roughly six years later. It turns out that when one spouse's level of activity increased from one occasion to the next, the other spouse tended to become more active as well.

The lesson here is to surround yourself with people who share your commitment to being active. And remember that peer pressure can work in the opposite direction, with sedentary partners, relatives, or friends dampening your motivation and even sabotaging your efforts to exercise ("forget the exercise, let's go eat!"). If you find yourself in this situation, don't brag about your exercise accomplishments to the inactive people around you, since this will only exacerbate the problem by making them feel annoyed and resentful. Instead, let them know that being healthy is important to you and that you want and need their support. And who knows—maybe your example will eventually get them off the couch.

members of fitness networks won't be annoyed when you revel in your latest exercise accomplishments.

CLAIM YOUR REWARD

Being rewarded for hard work can be a powerful incentive to continue. Consider giving yourself a gift when you reach a particular milestone, whether it's, say, increasing the intensity of your workout or going a month without missing a day of exercise. The reward should be something that you enjoy and don't routinely get, such as a massage, concert tickets, or a vacation. Just steer clear of food, especially if you're watching your weight. Rewarding yourself with a piece of cake or a large meal can easily become a habit and undermine your efforts.

Some companies offer financial incentives for their workers to exercise, an approach that research suggests can be effective. A review of 11 randomized studies collectively involving about 1,500 people concluded that using money as a reward makes recipients more likely to exercise and stick with it for up to six months and possibly longer.

How financial incentives are structured can influence their effectiveness. In one study, researchers gave 280 participants the goal of reaching 7,000 steps per day. Subjects were randomly assigned to one of four groups: People in the first group received $1.40 for every day the goal was achieved (which adds up to $42 a month). Those in the second group were eligible to win a lottery prize of $1.40 for each day the goal was achieved. Participants in the third group received $42 in an online bank account on the first day of every month, with $1.40 deducted each day they failed to reach the goal. The fourth group served as a control with no financial incentive.

After 13 weeks, the clear winner was the group that had received money up front. These participants achieved their daily goal 45 percent of the time, compared to only about 30 percent among subjects in the control group. What's notable is that the threat of "losing" $1.40 a day was a more powerful incentive than the promise of earning it. Scientists who study economics and decision theory call this phenomenon "loss aversion": As much as we love receiving money, we hate losing it even more.

So how can you apply these findings to increase your own motivation? One way is to give a certain amount of money each month to a trusted friend, relative, or colleague. If you reach your goal, you get the money back with the option of allocating it toward a reward such as a vacation. But if you fail to meet your goal, the other person keeps the money and gives it to a cause that you don't like. (For example, if you're a conservative Republican, they might donate it to the campaign of a liberal Democrat.) Draw up a contract that spells out the terms, including your goals, the length of the agreement, the amount of money involved, and what the other person should do with the money if you don't meet your objective.

You can also find websites or apps that take your money and give it to charity or other users who have achieved their goals if you fail to meet yours. However it's done, putting your own money at stake can be an effective motivator, according to research. In one study, employees of a large company who made fitness commitments backed by their own funds went to the gym 50 percent more often than those who didn't have this incentive.

Financial rewards are what psychologists call "extrinsic" motivation—an inducement that comes from the outside. This tends to work best as you're starting a workout program but typically becomes less effective over time. To make exercise a long-term habit, what we need is "intrinsic" motivation—an incentive that comes from within ourselves. Though it can take time, viewing exercise as something that we want to do is the most powerful motivator of all.

ADJUST YOUR ATTITUDE

Ask people to list words they associate with exercise, and what you often hear are variations on what I call the three "deadly D's": "dislike," "dread," and "drudgery." Too often we think of exercise as an unpleasant chore—something that we think we *should* do but don't really *want* to do. Perhaps those negative attitudes arise from an expectation of discomfort, pain, or boredom. Or from a fear of feeling self-conscious while working out. Or from past failed attempts to lose weight with exercise. Or from unpleasant childhood memories like those I described in chapter 1.

Whatever the case, negative beliefs about physical activity are sure-fire motivation-killers, and eliminating them is crucial for making exercise a

Is the drive to exercise genetic?

My mother likes to exercise. So did my father. His sister does too. Her daughter (my first cousin) is a personal trainer. And while my sister would tell you that she doesn't love working out, she's an avid exerciser as well. All of which makes me wonder whether I share a genetic makeup with these relatives that predisposes us to be active. Or is the explanation nurture rather than nature?

Experiments in lab animals offer hints that a tendency to exercise may be inborn. In one study, researchers placed rats in cages with running wheels and observed how much the animals voluntarily ran. The most active males were bred with the most active females. Ditto for the least active rats. Their offspring were bred in a similar fashion. The process continued through multiple generations.

In the end, the exercise-loving rats ran 10 times more than the lazy ones. Looking for possible explanations, the researchers found that the couch-potato rats weren't any fatter than the running rats. But there were several dozen genes that differed between the high and low runners, which suggests that the urge to exercise is genetic—at least in lab rats.

Human studies of twins provide more relevant evidence. If activity levels are more similar among pairs of identical twins (who share 100 percent of their genes) than pairs of fraternal twins (who share just 50 percent), this suggests that genetics play a role. And that in fact is what research overall has found. A study that looked at data from 37,000 twin pairs in seven countries concluded that 62 percent of the variation in exercise participation is due to heredity.

But there's no single "exercise gene." Instead, a variety of genetic traits such as personality, nervous system responses to exercise (which can dictate whether we feel pleasure or pain), and athletic ability probably have an impact. While these things may provide a nudge in one direction or another (or maybe in opposite directions simultaneously), they don't mean you're predestined to a life of activity or sloth. Ultimately, you have the power to decide.

AVOID OFF-RAMPS

permanent habit. In her book *No Sweat*, Michelle Segar, a motivation scientist at the University of Michigan, describes a process to rid ourselves of negative attitudes toward physical activity, or, in her words, to "exorcise" exercise. It involves writing down all the beliefs and expectations about exercise that undermine your desire to do it, and then tearing up the paper and throwing it away.

Try to replace these beliefs with positive ones about how physical activity enhances your life. This may include some of the immediate payoffs described at the beginning of this chapter, such as a better mood or more energy. Perhaps exercise makes you feel stronger (both physically and mentally), more empowered, or more in control of your life—or some combination of all these.

The key is to transform exercise from something that you *have* to do into something that you *want* to do. Or, as Segar puts it, from a chore into a gift. This process takes time and patience, but it's certainly worth the effort. Changing our attitude is the surest way to steer clear of the exercise off-ramps that we all encounter and to keep moving for a lifetime.

Gear Up

Without question, it's easier to spend money on fitness-related gear than to use that gear as intended. As evidence, look no further than everyone you know who wears tracksuits without ever setting foot on a track (or anyplace else to run or walk), or all those who own home gym equipment that collects cobwebs or serves as a clothes rack.

With so much fitness-related stuff for sale, it's easy to get lured by promises that a product will make you leaner, faster, stronger, or sexier. The truth, however, is that you don't need most of this gear to get or stay fit. All that's required for the *Fitter Faster* program is good shoes, comfortable clothes, and some basic equipment.

GOOD SOLES

The type of athletic shoes you need depends on your activities. If you're a walker, your shoes should be lightweight and have sufficient cushioning to make them comfortable. They should be relatively flexible, especially around the forefoot since we walk by pushing off with our toes.

A running shoe may be fine for walking, but a walking shoe is not appropriate for running. Running shoes typically have more cushioning than walking shoes to help absorb the greater force with which runners hit the ground. And since the mechanics of running differ from those of walking, running shoes often are most flexible at the arch or midfoot instead of the forefoot. In addition, good running shoes have a wide "toe box"—the area where your toes are—to accommodate the spread of your foot when it strikes the ground.

Beyond that, it gets more complicated—and controversial. Running shoes come in several categories, each designed for a different foot type: *Stability* shoes are for runners whose feet roll inward excessively or "overpronate" when they land; *motion control* shoes are intended for those who have flat feet and are severe overpronators; and *neutral* shoes are designed for runners with high arches who don't overpronate or who underpronate. If you've ever bought shoes at a running store, perhaps a salesperson there has analyzed your footprint or foot motion to determine which type of shoe is best for you.

For years it's been widely assumed that overpronation leads to injuries and that using the right shoe can reduce the risk. But research has called these beliefs into question. In a one-year study of more than 900 novice runners, all were instructed to use the same model of neutral shoes regardless of their foot type. Running distances were tracked with a GPS watch. It turns out that the runners with overpronated feet experienced fewer injuries than those with neutral feet, even though the overpronators were using the "wrong" shoe.

This study comes on the heels of research among military recruits, which showed that assigning shoes based on foot type did not reduce injury risk. While a stability or motion-control shoe may be optimal for some people, the best choice is likely a neutral shoe that's comfortable, according to researchers who reviewed the evidence. But step gingerly when it comes to heavily cushioned or "maximalist" shoes. It's possible that these may alter your running form and cause you to land with more force.

Then there's the other extreme: running barefoot or wearing "minimalist" shoes that are supposed to simulate going barefoot. A growing number of people, who see the practice as more natural, have adopted it as a way to reduce injuries, strengthen muscles, and improve performance. In fact, research does show that the biomechanics of running change when you shed your shoes. For example, experienced barefoot runners hit the ground with the midfoot or forefoot, while shod runners tend to strike with the heel. But whether these changes translate into benefits is unknown. And even if barefoot running does reduce the risk of some injuries, it may increase the risk of others, especially when you're a newbie. As a result, if you want to switch from conventional to minimalist shoes or bare feet, you should do so very gradually.

Some other unconventional shoes you may have encountered are so-called toning shoes. These have rounded soles, which create a feeling of instability as though you're walking on sand. Proponents claim that the shoes can, among other things, strengthen muscles, reduce joint pain, improve circulation, promote weight loss, and even get rid of cellulite. There's little solid science to support these assertions, however.

An independent study by the American Council on Exercise had subjects walk on a treadmill in toning shoes and conventional athletic shoes as heart rate, calorie burning, muscle activation, and other variables were measured. The researchers concluded that toning shoes did not help wearers "exercise more intensely, burn more calories, or improve muscle strength and tone." Some experts worry that the shoes may increase the risk of injuries and falling in some people.

A better option is a cross-trainer, which you can use for various *Fitter Faster* activities, including weightlifting and aerobic training. However, if you do a lot of running, you also need a pair of running shoes.

Whatever type of athletic shoe you're considering, the following tips can help you get the most out of your purchase:

- Don't assume that models with lots of fancy features are better. The same goes for shoes that are endorsed by celebrities or sell for the highest price. At the same time, don't skimp. Shoes are a key equipment purchase for physical activity, and they're the most important investment you'll make for activities such as walking and running.
- Buy late in the day. Our feet tend to expand throughout the day, and you want to get fitted when your feet are at their largest.
- Try shoes on with the socks you'll be wearing.
- Make sure there's space equal to the width of your thumb between your longest toe and the front of the shoe. You should be able to wiggle all your toes, and the heel should not slip.
- Walk around on different surfaces to make sure the shoes are comfortable.

- Don't wear your athletic shoes for everyday activities, since this will cause them to wear out faster. Save them for exercise or sports.
- Replace shoes after 300 to 500 miles of walking or running. If you're not sure how many miles you've covered, get new shoes every six to 12 months, depending on how frequently you use them.

KEEP YOUR COOL

For some people, workout clothing is all about looking good. But what really matters is that it makes you feel good—cool, comfortable, and not clammy. That's the promise of a plethora of lightweight athletic garments, from shirts and tights to socks and underwear. Typically these are made of synthetic fabrics such as polyester and Lycra, which pull (or wick) sweat from your skin to outer layers of the clothes, where the moisture evaporates. Cotton, on the other hand, absorbs moisture but doesn't promote evaporation. As a result, your shirt (or other clothing) can feel soaked and heavy after a workout.

A drawback of polyester is that it tends to stink more than cotton after exercise. In one study, researchers collected the sweaty shirts of 26 subjects after an hour of intensive spinning. The next day, trained sniffers determined that the polyester shirts smelled worse than the cotton ones. (It's unclear who exactly agreed to do this job or why.) Micrococci, a type of bacteria that break down sweat and cause unpleasant odor, were found to grow only on the polyester garments. That's important because sweat itself is generally odor-free; it's the combination of sweat and certain bacteria that literally raises a stink. (For more on sweating, see page 69.)

You can find "odor-resistant" synthetic fabrics, which are treated with various antibacterial compounds. Among the most common is silver, typically applied in tiny amounts known as nanoparticles. But some research suggests that silver-treated clothing may not work as well as promised to reduce bacteria and odor. What's more, a significant amount of the silver may come out in the wash, reducing the effectiveness of the garments and potentially harming the environment. There

DAN
AGE 45
CHICAGO, ILLINOIS

Dan's job as a cameraman for a local news station meant he was on his feet all day, much of the time while lugging TV production gear. On the advice of a fellow cameraman, Dan invested in some sturdy hiking boots so he would have greater ankle support. He found the boots to be extremely comfortable and wore them every day, often for over 15 hours. When his boots wore out, Dan replaced them with another pair and continued to do so for several years.

Although his job kept him busy, Dan made time for exercising at the gym, playing tennis, and biking with friends, all of which he enjoyed. But over time, these activities seemingly began to take a toll on his body. "I started feeling a lot of knee and back pain," Dan recalls. "It was enough that I stopped doing physical activity outside of work. It just hurt too much."

Visits to doctors revealed no significant injuries or strains, but his aches and pains continued to grow. And now they were accompanied by fatigue. All this was happening around the time he needed to replace his boots. Unable to find another of the same pair quickly, Dan laced up some running shoes and started wearing those to work instead. By the end of the first week, his back and knee pain were gone.

Dan did some research and spoke to a knowledgeable shoe salesman. What he learned surprised him: Back and other body pain can start in the feet. It turns out that Dan's pain wasn't due to exercise or the equipment on his back; it was caused by the shoes on his feet. Lugging equipment around in the wrong footwear had been taxing his body.

Now Dan wears lightweight running shoes for his job. He's free of pain and has resumed his workouts and other activities. "All it took was a good pair of shoes," he says, "to help me stay on my feet."

49

are also concerns that exposing our skin to silver nanoparticles may pose a health risk, though there's no direct evidence for this.

If you prefer something other than synthetic fabrics or cotton, there's wool—but not the type in itchy sweaters. Athletic apparel made of merino wool is lightweight, breathable, and appropriate for hot or cold conditions. It's more odor-resistant than polyester and doesn't get wet with sweat, as cotton does. The main downside is the relatively hefty price.

Other options include bamboo or blends of natural and synthetic materials. Whatever fabric you choose, make sure the clothing is comfortable and loose enough to allow easy movement. At the same time, it shouldn't be so loose that it gets in the way of your activity. (Long, baggy pants, for example, don't mix well with bike pedals or chains.) If you're exercising in the cold, dress in layers consisting of an inner layer that wicks moisture away from your skin, a middle layer (such as fleece or wool) that provides insulation, and an outer layer (such as a nylon jacket) that protects you from wind, snow, and rain. And of course don't forget your mother's advice to wear a hat and gloves.

SQUEEZE PLAY

Compression garments—those tight-fitting shirts, sleeves, shorts, socks, and other clothes—have become popular among elite athletes and average exercisers alike. Long used as a treatment for circulatory problems, compression clothing is touted as a way to boost athletic performance by increasing the flow of oxygenated blood to muscles.

While some research suggests that these garments may have small effects on high-intensity activities such as sprinting or vertical jumping, many other studies have shown no performance benefits. For example, a review of 32 studies in which subjects wore compression socks, tights, shorts, or calf sleeves while running a variety of distances (from 400 meters to marathons) found no effects overall on race times.

The evidence is stronger for another purported benefit: aiding recovery after exercise. Overall, research suggests that compression gear can reduce post-exercise muscle soreness and swelling, which may begin 12 to 24 hours following a workout and last for several days. There's a catch, however: To see results, you need to wear the clothing after you're through exercising, ideally for a couple of days. As one review of the evidence put it, "the longer an athlete can wear compression following exercise, the better." For many people, staying squeezed in compression clothes for prolonged periods may be just as unpleasant as the soreness that it's supposed to prevent. (For more on post-exercise soreness and how to reduce it, see chapter 9.)

If you like the way compression garments feel and look, keep wearing them. There's no harm in doing so, and they may enhance your workout if you believe they will. Placebos, it turns out, can provide a nice boost in our quest for fitness, just as they often do in other aspects of life.

DON'T PLAY DUMB

If you exercise at home and don't already own dumbbells, you'll need to purchase them for the *Fitter Faster* program. Basically, there are two types: conventional, and adjustable.

Conventional dumbbells come in fixed weights. For these you'll need multiple pairs. That's because different exercises require different-sized weights, and as you progress, you'll be able to lift heavier weights. Start with the lightest weight you think you'll need and buy a few pairs in 5-pound (or lighter) increments above that. Once you have a better sense of how much weight you're able to lift for each exercise, you can purchase additional weights.

Adjustable dumbbells, on the other hand, involve one pair of handles, to which you add or remove weight as needed. If you opt for adjustables, look for the kind that let you turn a dial or insert a pin to change the weight. You want to avoid adjustable dumbbells that require you to manually remove and add plates, a process that can be cumbersome and time-consuming. Our program is all about getting through your workout quickly, and you don't want to waste time fiddling with weights.

Some dumbbells are made of rubber; others of vinyl or metal. Further, the ends come in different shapes, including round (which roll) and hexagonal (which don't). The grips vary as well by material, texture, and circumference. Even if you plan to buy dumbbells online, it's a good idea to visit a sporting goods store and test weights to find a type that feels best to you. If you end up with dumbbells that you don't like, you're much less likely to use them.

When you're purchasing dumbbells, you may want to consider a few other pieces of equipment as well. While none is essential for the *Fitter Faster* plan, all of these can be useful.

Weight rack: A place to store your dumbbells will help you keep multiple sets organized. Also, by keeping the weights off the floor, a rack can save space and reduce your risk of tripping on them.

Gloves: A pair of weightlifting gloves can make handling weights more comfortable. Gloves improve your grip, preventing weights from slipping because of sweaty hands. And they protect you from blisters and calluses.

Weight bench: Some *Fitter Faster* exercises call for a couch or flat bench. If there's no couch in the area of your house where you work out, it's a good idea to add a bench. And even if you have a couch nearby, you may find a bench easier to use. Choose one that's sturdy and comfortable. It doesn't have to incline, though you may want this feature down the road as you advance in your exercise program.

Mat: With our program, you'll be doing some exercises on the floor; if the surface is hard, you'll need to add some cushioning. Though a thick towel or two can suffice, a nonslip mat with good padding can make the exercises more comfortable.

For information about two other popular pieces of home equipment, abdominal devices and foam rollers, see pages 85 and 92, respectively.

HEAVY MACHINERY

Home exercise equipment such as treadmills, elliptical machines, and stationary bikes aren't necessary for a fitness program. The *Fitter Faster* plan includes an array of options from hiking to dancing that don't require you to step on a machine if you prefer not to. Still, home equipment can make working out more convenient, especially if you have a demanding schedule or live in an area where you can't do outdoor activities year-round.

Does walking with weights enhance your workout?

Carrying small dumbbells or wearing wrist weights seems in theory like a good way to boost the intensity of your walks while also working your upper body. In fact, adding weight does burn more calories. But there's a problem: The light weights that people often use for walking typically burn too few extra calories to really matter. And heavier weights necessary for meaningful calorie burning may alter your natural arm swing and increase the risk of injuries to arms, shoulders, wrists, and elbows. In short, the downsides likely outweigh any benefits.

Ankle weights are not a good alternative because they increase susceptibility to lower-body injuries. Weighted vests are safer than ankle, wrist, or hand weights. To be effective, they should weigh 10 to 20 percent of your weight.

A better option is to walk with poles. The practice, sometimes called Nordic walking or exerstriding, originated in Finland as an off-season training method for cross-country skiers. Research suggests that pole-walking works upper-body and abdominal muscles, allows you to walk faster, and burns more calories than regular walking—all without making you feel as though you're working harder.

In addition, unlike weights, which may put stress on your joints, pole-walking takes pressure off your knees, hips, and lower back. It promotes good posture and can help improve balance and stability.

Techniques for Nordic walking and exerstriding vary somewhat, as do the poles used for each. Whichever you choose, make sure the poles feel comfortable and that you learn and use proper form.

Treadmills are the most popular type of home equipment, with lots of different options available. Among the most important considerations are sturdiness and cushioning, especially if you plan to run. In addition, the belt should be long enough to accommodate your stride and wide enough for your stance. Make sure the belt moves smoothly at all speeds and that the motor isn't too noisy. Non-motorized treadmills are less expensive but can be hard to get started and don't allow you to change the incline while you're moving. If you have limited space, a folding treadmill may be a good choice.

If you plan to use the treadmill for *Fitter Faster* interval training (which entails alternating between greater and lesser intensity), look for models that let you change the speed and incline quickly and easily during your workout. In addition, many treadmills include entertainment features ranging from iPod/iPhone docking stations to built-in televisions. If such bells and whistles increase your motivation to use the treadmill regularly, they may well be worth the extra cost. Otherwise, you can save money by going for a simpler model.

Don't skimp on safety, however. Treadmill-related injuries send tens of thousands of Americans to emergency rooms every year. The treadmill you choose should have an emergency stop button that's easily accessible and a shut-off safety key that attaches firmly to your clothing. In addition, you should be able to grab the safety rails easily and comfortably. Place the back of the machine at least six and a half feet away from walls, windows, and furniture, and leave 18 inches or more of free space on each side. (For more on preventing exercise-related injuries, see pages 127–131.)

Elliptical machines combine the movements of stair-stepping, biking, and cross-country skiing. Moderate effort on an elliptical burns fewer calories than running but more than walking on a treadmill with no incline at a relatively brisk pace of 3.5 miles per hour. An elliptical machine also puts less stress on joints.

The flywheel on an elliptical machine may be in the front, middle, or back. The placement can determine the smoothness and overall feel of the motion, so it's important to try different styles to see which you like best. As with a treadmill, the machine should feel sturdy and be able to accommodate your stride. In addition, the handles should be comfortable. For safety, be sure you have enough free space not only around the machine but also above it, since the pedals can put you a foot or two off the floor.

Stationary bikes come in two basic types: recumbent and upright. A recumbent bike provides support for your spine and can be a good option if you have back or balance problems. However, an upright bike works more muscles and generally burns more calories. Whichever you choose, seat comfort is paramount. In addition, the handlebars should be easy to reach and the resistance easy to adjust.

Other considerations for stationary bikes, as well as treadmills and elliptical machines, include the following:

Display: Display monitors should be easy to see and the controls simple to use and understand. Keep in mind that some readings, such as calories burned, may not be accurate.

Programming: Many models come with preset programs that automatically alter the intensity of your exercise. These can add variety and increase the effectiveness of your workout, but if you prefer to make such changes manually, don't pay extra for the programming feature. If your machine includes a program for the "fat burning zone," ignore it. (For more on this, see pages 67–68.)

Heart-rate monitors: Equipment often includes heart-rate sensors, some of which are more accurate than others. In some cases, the machine will automatically adjust exercise intensity based on your target heart rate. However, as you'll see in chapter 5, the formulas used to calculate maximum and target heart rate often yield inaccurate results. Consequently, we don't rely on heart-rate monitors in our workout program (though some people may need to wear the devices during exercise for medical purposes). For a description of other ways to gauge intensity, see pages 66–67.

Child safety: Children can be seriously or even fatally injured if they play around an exercise machine, even if it's turned off. Keep kids away from the equipment at all times. If possible, purchase a model that requires a passcode or has other child-safety features.

Is walking or running on a treadmill as effective as doing so outside?

For some people, exercising on a treadmill makes them feel like a hamster in a wheel: They keep moving and go nowhere. For others, the convenience, consistency, and climate-controlled conditions outweigh any downsides. In addition, a treadmill may be easier on joints than concrete or asphalt—a benefit especially for those with joint problems—because the belt has more give.

But a treadmill may give you a somewhat less intense workout. Because there's no wind resistance, you don't have to work quite as hard to walk or run as you would outside at the same pace. Increasing the incline slightly, to .5 or 1 percent (depending on how fast you go), may help compensate for this difference. Also, repeatedly altering the incline during your walk or run may more closely replicate the variations in outdoor terrain, though most treadmills don't let you go downhill.

Try to maintain a natural stride—not too short or too long—and use proper form, which includes standing up straight and looking forward, not down. (For more on correct walking and running form, see page 127.) Don't hold on to the front or side rails while you exercise; this gives leg and other muscles a partial free ride and reduces the number of calories you burn. In addition, holding on causes an unnatural gait and can increase the risk of injuries. If you have to use the rails for balance, touch them lightly but don't grip them. Better yet, reduce the speed or incline until you're comfortable with letting go.

Warranties: *Consumer Reports* recommends warranties of at least three years on parts and one year on labor. The publication also advises against buying extended warranties.

Returns: Make sure you can return the equipment if you don't like it. Find out what, if any, return costs you might incur, including shipping fees.

KEEP ON TRACKIN'

Fitbits and other wearable fitness trackers aren't just a way to look cool or show off that you exercise. The data they provide can serve as motivation to get off the couch and keep pushing yourself. Indeed, research suggests that using the devices increases levels of physical activity somewhat.

Despite their ubiquity, fitness trackers aren't essential for exercise, however. Nor are they right for everyone. Some people find the gadgets to be too much trouble or the data confusing. Others simply aren't comfortable with this type of technology. By one estimate, one in three people who own trackers abandon them within six months.

If you think that a tracker may enhance your fitness efforts, first consider how you'll be using it. If it's simply to count steps, for example, a basic device can suffice. But if you want to track, say, where you've been or how much you've climbed, you'll need a model with features that record location or altitude. In short, make sure the device you choose provides feedback that's important to you.

As for accuracy, research shows that trackers generally get step counts right for activities such as walking. (The same goes for smartphone apps that track physical activity.) But calorie counts are often off. In a study of four popular devices, two worn on the wrist and two on the hip, the trackers overestimated calories burned during walking and jogging, and underestimated calories burned during everyday activities like vacuuming and gardening. Readings for cycling and weightlifting appear to be especially prone to error. Still, calorie counts aren't entirely useless. An increase from one day to another for the same activity can indicate that you're upping the intensity.

Some trackers display activity data on the device; others require you

57

Are 10,000 steps a day really optimal?

Surveys show that very few Americans know how much exercise they're supposed to get. But many people are familiar with the advice to walk 10,000 steps a day. And it's not unusual to see followers of this directive constantly checking their Fitbits in hopes of achieving the magic number and then announcing it to everyone within earshot when they do.

Certainly anything that gets people to move more is laudable. But it turns out that the 10,000-steps-a-day guideline is overly simplistic and based more on marketing than sound science. The concept originated in the 1960s with a Japanese manufacturer of a pedometer called *manpo-kei*, which translates to "10,000 steps meter." It's thought that the number 10,000 was chosen because of its exalted status in Japanese culture.

What research shows is that getting fewer than 5,000 steps a day equates to being sedentary and that adding 3,000 to this baseline, for a total of 8,000 steps, is enough to meet the standard exercise recommendations for healthy adults. But there are two key requirements: 1) the 3,000 additional steps need to be taken at a relatively brisk pace of at least 100 per minute; and 2) they need to be done in increments of at least 10 minutes.

If you don't meet both of these conditions, you could be falling short, even if you get to 10,000 steps. For example, in a study of people who had osteoarthritis of the knee or were at high risk for it, more than 75 percent of those who walked at least 10,000 steps a day failed to meet the exercise guidelines.

On the other hand, if you walk briskly and in spurts of 10 minutes or longer, fewer than 10,000 steps may suffice. Whatever the number, try to increase it by setting progressively higher goals for yourself. And for extra credit, use stairs whenever possible. Whether you're going up or down, you burn more calories per minute than by walking on flat ground.

to use an app to access the information. Whatever the case, it should be presented in a fashion that's understandable and useful for you.

If you want additional ways to use or analyze the data, find out whether the tracker is compatible with other apps or devices that are of interest to you. If sharing data or doing fitness challenges with friends helps motivate you, look for social networking features that you like. The more that a tracker meets your specific needs, the more likely it will stay on your body rather than in a drawer.

Get Smart

What You Need to Know About Aerobic Exercise, Strength Training, and Stretching

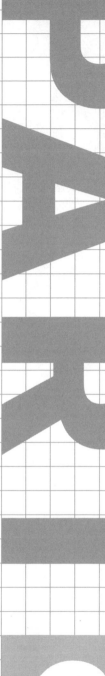

PART 2

Take It
to Heart

There once was a time when the sight of someone running past your house was so rare that you might have assumed the person to be either crazy or an escapee from the law (or an angry spouse). That changed in 1968 with the publication of the best-selling book *Aerobics* by fitness pioneer Dr. Kenneth Cooper, in which he introduced the concept of aerobic exercise. Today, his once-revolutionary ideas about exercise are universally embraced, and it's unusual *not* to see joggers out on any given day.

The term "aerobic"—Cooper added the "s" and coined the word "aerobics"—means "with oxygen." Also known as cardio or endurance exercise, aerobic activities work large muscle groups continuously and rhythmically at an intensity that can be sustained. The heart beats faster to deliver enough oxygen-rich blood to muscles, which use the oxygen to burn carbohydrates and fat for fuel. (In contrast, anaerobic exercises such as sprinting or heavy weightlifting, which are done in short, intense bursts, don't depend on oxygen.)

Doing aerobic exercise regularly leads to a number of beneficial changes in the body: The heart becomes stronger and is able to pump more blood with each beat. Resting heart rate decreases. Blood vessels expand and remain flexible. Muscles are better able to use oxygen from the blood. Mitochondria (the powerhouses of cells) in muscle increase in number, size, and activity, the result of which is an improved ability to burn fat and carbohydrates for energy.

Taken together, these and other changes add up to improved cardiovascular (or cardiorespiratory) fitness. And better cardiovascular fitness appears to be largely responsible for many of the health benefits of exercise, from decreased heart-attack risk to increased brain volume.

To achieve these benefits, the Centers for Disease Control and Prevention, along with major health groups, recommends at least 30 minutes a day, five days a week, of moderate-intensity aerobic activities. It's okay to break up the activities into bouts as short as 10 minutes, as long as they add up to the recommended totals. These levels, while good for your health, aren't typically enough to control weight. For that, you may need twice the recommended amount of exercise – or more.

Thirty or 60 minutes a day is a bigger time commitment than many of us are able or willing to make. Later in this chapter, I'll explain how the *Fitter Faster* program allows you to spend just a fraction of that on aerobic exercise and see benefits that are the same or even greater. But first I'll discuss how to gauge the intensity of your exercise—something that's crucial for short workouts to be effective.

MEET THE METS

Exercise scientists often gauge intensity using METs, which does not refer to players on a certain Major League Baseball team. (So if you're a Phillies or Yankees fan, you can keep reading.) METs, which stand for **m**etabolic **e**quivalents of **t**ask, measure how much energy you expend (expressed in calories) at a particular activity compared to what you expend at rest. One MET is your resting metabolic rate, meaning the rate at which you burn calories while sitting quietly. An activity of 3 METs, for example, would burn three times as many calories as you would at rest; a 6-MET activity would burn six times as many calories.

Moderate-intensity aerobic activities have METs of 3.0 to 5.9. Recreational activities such as brisk walking, doubles tennis, ballroom dancing, and biking (slower than 10 miles per hour) fall into this category. So do chores such as mopping, sweeping, vacuuming, mowing the lawn,

RICHARD

AGE 50

RANDOLPH, NEW JERSEY

For Richard, who grew up in an Italian family, food was always an important part of his life. To counteract the effects of pasta and pastries, he tried to stay active, though with mixed success. During a medical checkup in his mid-40s, Richard got some disconcerting news: He was prediabetic and had high blood pressure, for which He would need to take medication.

After the shock wore off, Richard set about changing his lifestyle by eliminating many of the foods he'd been eating his entire life. But he knew that diet alone wasn't enough to improve his cardiovascular health. Richard would need to incorporate more aerobic exercise into his daily routine, which included a 75-minute one-way commute to a demanding job. Hitting the gym felt like a chore, however. Richard realized that if he was going to be active and stick with it, he would have to do something that he enjoyed and that kept him around other people.

Eventually he found it: ice hockey, which had been his favorite sport when he was young. "Skating for me was as close to flying as I could get without leaving the ground," he says. "The movement together with the game brought me pure joy."

Richard now works out on the ice two or three times a week, playing on a recreation-league hockey team. The aerobic workout that it provides, along with yoga and changes in his diet, has helped Richard successfully manage his prediabetes and high blood pressure. He has shed 50 pounds and no longer needs medication. "Exercise was the key," he says, "and there's no downside. I'm more fit and having fun."

and raking leaves. More enjoyable everyday activities like playing with children or pets qualify as well. (I'm sorry to report that sexual activity, even if it's, uh, strenuous, doesn't make the cut.)

Vigorous activities are those with METs of 6 or more. Included are jogging, jumping rope, swimming laps, playing singles tennis, shoveling snow, and carrying boxes or furniture up stairs.

An alternative for assessing intensity is the so-called rating of perceived exertion, or RPE. Basically, this is a scale that measures how hard you feel your body is working overall. The traditional version, known as the Borg scale, goes from 6 (no exertion) to 20 (maximum exertion). A rating of 11 to 14 corresponds to moderate-intensity exercise, while 15 to 18 means the activity is vigorous.

While there's a rationale behind this seemingly random scale—each number multiplied by 10 correlates with your heart rate at that level of activity—figuring out where exactly you fall between 6 and 20 can be tricky. A more intuitive RPE scale goes from 1 to 10, with a 5 or 6 indicating moderate-intensity exercise and 7 or 8 vigorous activity.

Perhaps the easiest way to tell how hard you're working is the talk test. If you can talk and sing during your activity without becoming breathless, the intensity level is low. If you can talk but *not* sing, the intensity is moderate. And if you can say only a few words before having to catch your breath, you're doing vigorous exercise.

(DON'T) DO THE MATH

Another way of assessing aerobic intensity is to measure your heart rate. Some group exercise programs have participants wear heart-rate monitors and stay within a particular training zone, while many gyms and cardio machines display charts showing what your target heart rate should be.

Exercise done at 50 to 70 percent of your maximum heart rate (MHR) is considered moderately intense, with the lower end of the range intended for people who are beginners or out of shape. Activities that put you at 70 to 85 percent of MHR qualify as vigorous.

That's the straightforward part. How to measure MHR gets complicated, though. The conventional (and easiest) way is to subtract your age from 220. But that formula, based on studies from the 1970s in mainly young and middle-aged men, is too simplistic and often yields inaccurate results, especially in older people.

Still, many gyms, coaches, personal trainers, and fitness websites continue to recommend this method, which may lead some people to under-exert themselves and others to overdo it.

An alternative formula developed by researchers at the University of Colorado is to multiply your age by .7 and subtract that number from 208. But other researchers have found this method to be lacking as well. Another formula is to take 64 percent of your age and subtract it from 211. Still others, developed by doctors at the Mayo Clinic, involve different calculations for men and women: 216 minus 93 percent of your age if you're male and 200 less 67 percent of your age if you're female. But only if you're 40 or over.

Got that?

Because of the complexity and shortcomings of these formulas, we don't rely on heart-rate monitoring in the *Fitter Faster* plan. (People with medical conditions may need to do so, however.) Instead, we suggest using the 10-point RPE scale or the talk test, both of which are relatively accurate and simple ways to gauge intensity.

Slow Burn

While we're on the subject of confusing computations, consider the issue of the "fat-burning" zone. This is the heart-rate range, displayed on charts in gyms and on cardio equipment, that's supposedly optimal for weight loss.

The target, which is 50 to 60 percent of MHR, is on the low end of the moderate-intensity zone. Go above that range, we're told, and get diminishing returns. In other words, exert less effort and lose more fat.

Sounds great. Unfortunately, it's not true.

When we exercise, our muscles can use stored fat or carbohydrates for fuel. How much of each depends on how vigorous the exercise is. If you work out at a lower intensity—for example, walking at a somewhat leisurely pace—most of the calories you burn will come from fat. Step it up to a run, and the percentage of calories from fat goes down, while the percentage from carbs goes up.

Though this sounds as though walking is better than running, the catch is that running burns more calories overall. For instance, someone weighing 150 pounds who walked at a pace of 3 miles per hour for 30 minutes would burn about 120 calories. Eighty percent of those calories, or 96, might come from fat.

If that person were to run at a 10-minute-mile pace (i.e., 6 miles per hour) for 30 minutes, the number of calories burned would be roughly 350. Even though a lower percentage of calories—say half—would come from fat, this still adds up to 175 fat calories, which is greater than the number burned by walking for the same length of time.

Now if the same person walked for an hour, they might burn more fat calories than if they ran for 30 minutes, but they would still burn *fewer* total calories.

The takeaway from all this number-crunching is that calorie-burning is a function of time *and* intensity. This means that the less vigorously you're able or willing to work out, the more time you need to put in for optimal results. On the flip side, the more vigorously you're able to exercise, the less time you need to spend—a key principle behind the *Fitter Faster* program.

HIIT YOUR STRIDE

If someone said they could show you how to do as little as five minutes of exercise and get the same aerobic benefits that you would from a standard 45-minute workout, you might suspect you were being scammed. But in fact, a growing body of research suggests that so-called high-intensity interval training, or HIIT for short, can greatly reduce the amount of time you need to exercise while increasing cardiorespiratory fitness as much as conventional moderate-intensity exercise does, if not more so.

A crucial part of the *Fitter Faster* program, HIIT involves alternating short spurts of intense exercise with periods of light exercise or rest. You go hard, then easy, hard, then easy, and so on, as opposed to exercising at the same intensity for, say, 30 minutes—as you would with a conventional aerobic workout. A wide array of exercises can be adapted to HIIT, including walking, running, swimming, rowing, stair-climbing,

Does more sweating mean a more intense workout?

Ifeel sorry for anyone who uses the treadmill after me at my gym. Despite my best efforts to wipe it down when I'm done, the unlucky soul is likely to touch, step in, or otherwise encounter one of the many pools of sweat that I typically deposit on the machine.

At the same time, I long regarded my profuse sweating with some degree of satisfaction because I saw it as evidence of how hard I was pushing myself. But it turns out I was wrong: How much you sweat doesn't necessarily correlate with how intense your workout is or how many calories you burn.

When your body temperature rises, your eccrine glands secrete sweat, and the evaporation of moisture from your skin helps you cool off. (Of course, sweating can occur for other reasons, such as stress or fear. That type of sweat comes from the apocrine glands, which are located mainly in the underarm and groin.)

How much we sweat during exercise is due to a number of factors, including gender (men tend to sweat more than women) and age (younger people sweat more than older people), as well as genetics, temperature, and humidity. Weight plays a role as well. Larger people tend to sweat more because their bodies generate more heat.

Another contributor is fitness level. Surprisingly, fit people tend to sweat sooner during exercise and more copiously than those who are less fit. Research suggests that as your fitness level improves, your body's heat-regulating system becomes more efficient, cooling you down faster and allowing you to work harder.

Don't be misled by the loss of a few pounds after a high-sweat workout. This is simply water weight that you gain back when you rehydrate and doesn't necessarily mean you've burned lots of calories.

On the flip side, don't assume that a low-sweat workout means you aren't working hard enough or burning enough calories. It could be that your sweat evaporates quickly because you're exercising in air conditioning, near a fan, or outdoors on a windy day. Or, unlike me, you simply may not sweat much. Whatever the case, don't sweat it.

TAKE IT TO HEART

stationary cycling, doing calisthenics, or using an elliptical machine, any of which you can do for *Fitter Faster* workouts.

The HIIT routine often used in studies requires pedaling as hard as you can for 30 seconds on a stationary bike with the resistance level set very high. That's followed by four minutes of light cycling or rest. This regimen, known as the Wingate test, is done four to six times.

Other versions vary in the length of the high-intensity period (from less than 10 seconds to several minutes) as well as the level of intensity, the length of the recovery period, and the number of repetitions.

For example, a regimen developed by Martin Gibala, an exercise scientist at McMaster University who has extensively studied HIIT, includes one-minute, high-intensity bursts (at 9 on a perceived intensity scale of 10) interspersed with one-minute, low-intensity periods. The high-intensity intervals are done a total of 10 times.

A type of HIIT training known as Tabata, named for the Japanese researcher who developed it, involves going all-out for 20 seconds, resting for 10 seconds, and repeating seven more times.

Yet another HIIT variation known as the 7-Minute Workout, which was popularized by a 2013 *New York Times* article, combines cardio and strength training. The original version of this routine includes 12 different body-weight exercises such as push-ups, squats, and jumping jacks, done for 30 seconds each, with 10 seconds of rest between them.

The list goes on.

The concept behind HIIT isn't new. Athletes have long used interval training to improve performance. In the 1930s, for example, Swedish cross-country runners trained by sprinting toward a landmark such as a tree, then running more slowly, then speeding toward another landmark. This type of unstructured interval training, which continues to be used today, has a name sure to prompt snickering among seven-year-olds (and in some cases their parents too): *fartlek*, which means "speed play" in Swedish.

In recent years, researchers have conducted a number of studies on the health benefits of HIIT. Though most of the trials to date have been relatively small and short term, the evidence as a whole looks quite promising. Take, for example, the effect on cardiovascular fitness as measured by VO2 max, which is the maximum amount of oxygen the body can use during exercise. A review of trials concluded that HIIT increases VO2 max more than continuous aerobic exercise does.

Other research shows that HIIT can improve blood pressure, cholesterol levels, blood-sugar regulation, and blood-vessel function at least as well as continuous exercise. And HIIT may be more effective than conventional aerobic exercise at reducing so-called subcutaneous fat (the type right under the skin) as well as excess belly fat, which is considered especially harmful.

It's not completely clear why short bursts of exercise have such large effects. One possible reason is that HIIT activates so-called slow-twitch muscle fibers as well as fast-twitch fibers, which we use for quick, explosive movements. By contrast, conventional endurance exercise recruits mainly just slow-twitch fibers.

While most of the studies on HIIT have been in relatively young, healthy people, research suggests it's effective for middle-aged and older people as well. A study by Japanese researchers, for example, randomly assigned participants (average age 63) to do at least four days a week of either continuous moderate-intensity walking or interval walking (consisting of three minutes of easy walking, alternating with three minutes of fast walking, done five times). After five months, the HIIT walkers had greater improvements in VO2 peak (a measure similar to VO2 max) and blood pressure than the continuous walkers.

Likewise, HIIT can be beneficial for those with chronic conditions. A review of 10 studies involving people who were obese or suffering from heart disease, heart failure, high blood pressure, or metabolic syndrome (which is a combination of high blood pressure, high blood sugar, abnormal cholesterol, and excess belly fat) found that HIIT increased VO2 peak nearly two times more than continuous moderate aerobic exercise did. Other research shows that in people who have type 2 diabetes or are at increased risk for the condition, HIIT is superior to continuous exercise at reducing blood glucose levels.

Though high-intensity exercise may seem risky for people with heart disease or other chronic illnesses, studies have found that it's generally safe. However, those with chronic conditions should get clearance from their doctor before starting HIIT and do the workouts under professional supervision. If you're healthy but sedentary, it's also a good idea to check with your doctor before jumping into a HIIT exercise program.

71

Time Flies

The amount of time required to achieve benefits with HIIT is remarkably small. A study by Martin Gibala and his colleagues, for example, showed that a total of just 60 seconds of strenuous exercise—done in three 20-second intervals of "all-out" cycling, interspersed with two minutes of easy cycling—improved various measures of cardiovascular fitness in sedentary men as much as 45 minutes of continuous cycling at a moderately intense pace. The entire HIIT workout, which was done three times a week for 12 weeks, lasted only 10 minutes with warm-up and cool-down.

Likewise, research in young, physically active women found that a Tabata-style workout lasting just under four minutes increased VO2 peak as much as running continuously on a treadmill for 30 minutes. In each session, the HIIT subjects performed as many repetitions as possible of exercises such as jumping jacks, mountain climbers, or burpees (more on what these are in chapter 10) for 20 seconds. This was done eight times, with 10 seconds of rest between intervals. With four sessions per week, the HIIT participants exercised a total of about 15 minutes a week, compared to two hours for the treadmill runners.

Of course, shorter workouts offer no real advantage if they're so unpleasant that you don't do them. The key here appears to be the type of HIIT regimen. While some research shows that people react negatively to very arduous forms such as the Wingate test, studies also find that exercisers like other HIIT regimens.

For example, a study of 44 inactive adults assigned the subjects to do three workouts: continuous moderate-intensity cycling for 40 minutes; continuous vigorous cycling for 20 minutes; and a HIIT regimen for 20 minutes, consisting of 60-second high-intensity intervals interspersed with 60-second low-intensity intervals. A majority of participants said that they most preferred HIIT.

One reason may be that doing HIIT, at least certain versions that don't require all-out effort, makes people feel that they're exerting less effort overall than when doing continuous exercise. Those 20-, 30-, or 60-second high-intensity intervals are unpleasant, but the fact that they're relatively short and broken up by rest periods makes the exercise tolerable. In a study of subjects who were unfit and overweight, they reported lower ratings of perceived exertion after a HIIT workout consisting of 30-second intervals than they did after a 20-minute vigorous workout. (That was not the case, however, for HIIT workouts with two-minute intervals.)

Another factor is less drudgery: Breaking up exercise into intervals can be less boring than, say, walking on a treadmill at the same pace for 30 minutes and help make the time pass more quickly. That, combined with the lower time requirement, may increase the odds that you'll stick with HIIT. Indeed, in one study, researchers found that people with pre-diabetes, when exercising on their own for a month, were more likely to adhere to a HIIT regimen (consisting of 60-second intervals) than to continuous moderate-intensity exercise.

YOUR MILEAGE MAY VARY

If you've ever participated in a group exercise class, you've likely witnessed a potentially disconcerting truth about aerobic training: Not everyone responds the same. Some people quickly get more fit, while others struggle to make gains despite their best efforts. If you find yourself in the latter category, it can be quite frustrating.

Understanding this variation is the mission of a long-running research effort known as the HERITAGE Family Study. Putting more than 600 participants through a 20-week aerobic training program (consisting of cycling for 30 to 50 minutes, three times a week), the researchers found that the average increase in VO2 max was 17 percent. But the range of responses was wide, with some people experiencing increases as great as 56 percent and others seeing no improvement at all.

Variables such as age, gender, race, and initial fitness level don't appear to explain these differences. But the researchers have discovered that people within the same family are more likely to respond similarly to training than people from different families. What this suggests is that genetics plays a role. By the researchers' estimates, as much as half of the variation in responses to aerobic exercise is due to heredity.

Regardless of your genetics, though, increasing the intensity of your workouts can make your body more responsive to exercise. It's yet another reason why we've incorporated high-intensity intervals into the *Fitter Faster* plan. As you'll see in chapter 10, our program includes different HIIT regimens to add variety and different levels of difficulty so

Does fasting before aerobic exercise burn more fat?

So-called fasted cardio, which is aerobic exercise done on an empty stomach (typically first thing in the morning), has long been used by bodybuilders as a way to decrease body fat before a competition. Recently it has gained popularity among other exercisers looking to get leaner.

As previously mentioned, our bodies use stored carbohydrates (in the form of glycogen) or fat for fuel when we exercise. The rationale behind fasted cardio is that when glycogen stores are depleted because we haven't eaten, our bodies burn mainly fat. In addition, when insulin levels are low, which is the case when we fast, we burn more fat. But research overall has failed to prove that fasted cardio has an effect on body composition.

For example, in a four-week trial that randomly assigned young women to either fast or drink a 250-calorie shake before their aerobic workouts (while otherwise eating a low-calorie diet), both groups lost the same amount of fat and weight. Similarly, a study involving overweight women who did HIIT workouts for six weeks after either fasting or eating found no differences in fat loss.

A related claim is that when endurance athletes train in a fasted state, their performances during competitions (when they don't fast) improve. Think of it as doing practice runs in cement-lined shoes so you can go faster on race day. While research suggests that fasted cardio leads to metabolic adaptations that could in theory enhance performance, there's little evidence that they actually do.

But we do know that in people who aren't trained athletes, doing aerobic exercise—especially if it's vigorous—first thing on an empty stomach can be like driving your car on empty: You may not make it very far. Eating a light meal beforehand can keep your engine running. (For more on what to eat before, during, and after exercise, see chapter 8.)

that you can continue challenging yourself as you become more fit. The plan also includes conventional aerobic exercise since that's the type that large, long-term studies have linked to health benefits. (Such studies haven't yet been conducted on HIIT.) In short, our hybrid approach gives you the best of both, while significantly reducing the time spent on aerobic exercise.

Muscle In

If you'd asked me 20 years ago what I thought about weight training, I probably would have invoked Hans and Franz from the old *Saturday Night Live* skits. The buffoonish characters, who struck bodybuilder poses in their padded sweatsuits and derided those with flabby physiques as "girlie men," were a spoof of Arnold Schwarzenegger and bodybuilding culture.

Weight training, I thought, was for athletes, bodybuilders, and muscle heads—not regular people. But time and science have proven me wrong. Today you can find me in the gym several times a week, lifting weights alongside men and women of all ages, shapes, and sizes.

Weight training, also known as strength training or resistance training, is a crucial part of a well-rounded exercise program for everyone. Like aerobic exercise, it has been shown to improve cardiovascular health and help control blood sugar. As discussed in chapter 2, it can also help keep bones strong.

Unlike aerobic exercise, strength training can slow or reverse the loss of muscle mass that begins at age 30 and limits people's ability to do everyday activities as they get older. Muscle loss may also occur if you're shedding pounds on a calorie-restricted diet, and strength training can allow you to lose fat while preserving (and even increasing) muscle.

An increase in muscle mass can enhance your appearance by giving you greater muscle definition. But women need not fear that lifting

What's the best way to measure body fat?

Let's start with a method that's not reliable: weighing yourself. If you're doing resistance training, you may be adding muscle weight, which a scale can't tell you. Say, for example, that you've lost five pounds. This theoretically could mean that you've shed seven pounds of fat and gained two pounds of muscle. Or it could mean you've lost both three pounds of fat and two pounds of muscle. Either way, if your goal is to lose fat, the number on the scale would be deceiving.

Body mass index, or BMI, which is based on height and weight, also fails to distinguish between muscle and fat. As a result, someone who's muscular and athletic may have a high BMI (falsely categorizing him or her as "overweight" or "obese"), while a person with relatively high body fat and low muscle mass may fall in the "normal" range.

A better alternative may be to measure your waist circumference with a tape measure placed just above your hipbones. A reading of over 35 inches in women and 40 inches in men indicates excess belly fat, which is thought to be especially harmful.

Methods used to calculate the percentage of fat and lean tissue require special equipment. Here's the lowdown on four popular options:

- **Bioelectrical Impedance:** You stand on a platform or hold a device that sends an imperceptible electrical current through your body. Advantages: Easy, convenient. Disadvantage: Limited accuracy.
- **Skin Pinch:** Calipers are used to measure skinfold thickness in various areas of your body. Advantages: Convenient, inexpensive. Disadvantage: Accuracy varies depending on the tester's skill.
- **Underwater Weighing:** After blowing all the air out of your lungs, you're weighed while submerged in a tank of water. Advantage: Extremely accurate. Disadvantage: Inconvenient.
- **DEXA Scan:** You lie on a table while a machine emits low-energy X-rays. Advantages: Gold standard, shows location of fat in your body. Disadvantages: Can be expensive, not widely available.

78

weights will make them look like bulked-up bodybuilders. That requires higher levels of testosterone than women typically have.

What's more, there's evidence that strength training can help decrease body fat, though studies overall suggest that aerobic exercise is more effective. Your best bet may be a combination of resistance and aerobic training, which in some research has led to greater fat loss than either type of exercise alone.

Because of all these benefits, strength training plays a prominent role in the *Fitter Faster* program. And, as I'll explain later in this chapter, our approach allows you to get better results with shorter workouts. First, it's important to understand some basics about strength training.

TRY TO RESIST

A strength-training program should target all the major muscle groups: chest, back, shoulders, arms (including biceps and triceps), abdominals, and legs (quadriceps, hamstrings, and calves). The idea is to work the muscles against resistance, which typically comes from weights, weight machines, resistance bands, or your own body weight.

The aim of strength training, as strange as it may sound, is to cause tiny injuries (known as micro-tears) to your muscles. In response, so-called satellite cells in the muscles kick into action and fuse to muscle fibers to repair the damage and form new muscle protein. The result is greater strength and size. Enhanced nerve activity in response to resistance training also contributes to increased strength as well as athletic performance. What's more, resistance training strengthens ligaments (which attach bones to each other, stabilizing joints) and tendons (which attach muscles to bone, enabling bones to move).

To see such effects, healthy people are typically advised to do 8 to 12 reps when working with weights. ("Reps," short for repetitions, refers to the number of times in a row that you do the exercise.) Doing more reps (15 or 20) at a lighter weight can enhance muscle endurance, which is the ability of muscles to contract repeatedly over a sustained period. This is important for sports such as running or cycling that involve repetitive movements and for everyday activities. Higher rep counts at lower weights are also appropriate for beginners and older people.

Conversely, the conventional wisdom, backed by some studies, is that doing fewer reps with a heavy weight is best for maximizing strength. But other research finds that the number of reps and the size of the weight generally don't matter. Instead, what seems to be most important is working to muscle failure, which means continuing to lift the weight until you can't do another rep.

Regardless of how many reps you do, sticking with the same number at every workout can limit your progress. That's because our muscles adapt, and improvements slow down or stop. One way to avoid this is through what's known as periodization, which is varying the number of reps or other aspects of your routine according to a particular schedule. Overall, research shows that this can enhance results.

Increasing the weight as you become stronger is crucial. Too often, people plateau because they continue to use the same weight even after it's become relatively easy to lift. Another gain-limiting mistake is doing the same exercises at every workout, week after week, month after month. Incorporating different exercises into your workout regimen—and ones that are more challenging as you advance—will help ensure that you continue to make gains. And it will keep you from getting bored with the same routine.

As you'll see in chapter 10, the *Fitter Faster* program includes variations in the number of reps you do, the heaviness of the weights you use, and the exercises you perform so that you'll be able to maximize your results.

You'll also find that there aren't back-to-back weight-lifting days in our plan. The standard advice is to wait at least 48 hours between full-body strength-training sessions to allow time for muscles to recover. However, working the same muscles two days in a row may be fine for some people, depending on what exercises they do and how quickly their bodies recover. In any event, there's agreement that if you exercise different muscle groups on different days—say, upper body one day and lower body another—it's okay to work out on consecutive days.

UP TO SPEED

When it comes to how quickly you should raise and lower weights, a moderate speed is considered 1 to 2 seconds lifting (known as the concentric phase of the exercise) and 2 to 3 seconds lowering the weight

Can restricting blood flow during resistance exercise improve results?

Its nickname, "tourniquet training," makes it sound seedy or scary, if not both. But a growing number of athletes, from Olympic skiers to sumo wrestlers, swear by the technique formally known as blood flow restriction (BFR) exercise. The idea, which originated in Japan, is to partially restrict blood flow into the muscle and block the flow out while you lift weights. A version called Kaatsu uses computer-controlled cuffs placed around arms or legs during workouts. But non-automated cuffs or simple elastic wraps can also work.

BFR purportedly allows people to get bigger and stronger with relatively light weights—an advantage especially for those who can't use heavier weights because they're older, injured, or recovering from surgery. The technique is also touted as an adjunct to conventional weight training in athletes and other healthy people.

Though the evidence is limited, a review of studies has found that weight training with BFR appears to increase muscle size and strength more than an identical regimen without BFR. Scientists aren't sure why, but they suspect that reduced oxygen to muscles and increased swelling of muscle cells, among other things, lead to adaptations.

As you might expect, BFR has potential risks, especially if the cuff or wrap is too tight. These include bruising and numbness and, more seriously, blood clots. People with a history of vascular conditions such as deep vein thrombosis or varicose veins should avoid BFR. And those with high blood pressure or heart disease should proceed with extra caution.

If you're interested in trying BFR, it's best to work with a professional who is familiar with the technique and can make certain that you do it correctly and safely.

(the eccentric phase). But some people swear by slow-speed weight-training, in which the concentric and eccentric phases each last as long as 10 seconds. While a few studies suggest that this approach can produce superior strength gains, going that slowly can be extremely tedious and hard to do correctly without supervision. Hence, we do not include slow training in the *Fitter Faster* program.

On the flip side is fast lifting, which entails a concentric phase of less than 1 second and a moderate-speed eccentric phase. This increases power, which is related to strength but somewhat different. Strength is the ability to generate a force, while power refers to the rate at which force is exerted. Or, to use the technical definition, force times velocity. If strength is about lifting a boulder, power is about heaving it through the air.

Power is crucial for performance in sports ranging from golf to football. But it's also important for doing everyday activities such as climbing stairs or getting up from a chair. As we get older, the loss of power can contribute greatly to disability and feebleness. Therefore, a strength-training program ideally should include exercises for power even if you're not an athlete. Several trials in older people have shown that fast lifting results in greater improvements in physical functioning than does conventional strength training.

Another power-building approach is plyometrics, which are rapidly repeated jumping exercises. Examples include jumping rope, hops, squat jumps, tuck jumps, and burpees—all of which you'll find in the *Fitter Faster* workout program.

Besides working your muscles, plyometric exercises can get your heart rate up and provide an aerobic workout. In addition, research suggests that they may be especially beneficial for maintaining and building bone. In short, they're a great multipurpose exercise that can increase the efficiency of your workout by making it do double (or triple) duty. However, because plyometrics put stress on joints, they aren't a good option if you have arthritis or other joint-related problems.

HARD CORE

When many people hear the word "core," they think of abdominal muscles. But in fact a strong core is about much more than those six-pack

DOTTIE

AGE 82
JACKSONVILLE, FLORIDA

Growing up, Dottie chased her twin brother everywhere he went. But when he reached the door of the weight room, she was shut out. "In the 1950s, girls weren't allowed in the high school weight room," Dottie recalls. "So even though I was very active in sports, I never lifted weights when I was younger."

Two decades later, as she struggled during a run with her son, Dottie decided she wanted to increase her fitness level. She added weight lifting to her regimen and didn't let anything stop her. Even when she broke her collarbone, she kept working out. "I could still use my legs," she says. Her persistence has paid off: Dottie did triathlons well into her 70s, when she also set the world record in indoor rowing for her age group.

Strength training remains an important part of this octogenarian's routine. Dottie visits the gym two or three times a week, and when she can't get to the weights and bands she uses for training, she improvises. "Push-ups and sit-ups are the easiest thing to do anywhere, and if a hotel has phone books, I use those as weights," she says. Dottie believes that regular resistance training has helped prevent injuries and debilitation by maintaining her muscle strength and bone density.

When not in the gym, she finds other ways to stay fit. She squeezes balls to keep her hands strong, takes stairs instead of elevators in parking garages, and does yoga to maintain flexibility.

An inspiration to her friends, Dottie helps them find ways to improve their quality of life by getting stronger. She suggests they lift cans for arm strength and use old neckties to do stretching. "My friends say to me, 'I can't do what you do, Dottie,' and I tell them, 'maybe not. But you can do *something*.'"

abs you see in fitness magazines and occasionally in real life. Though definitions vary, your core generally refers to the muscles and connective tissue from the diaphragm down to the hips. Together these act like a corset, encircling the body to stabilize the spine and pelvis.

Whether you're bending, twisting, standing, or sitting, you rely on your core. It comes into play for not only recreational activities like golf, tennis, and running, but also everyday tasks such as picking up objects, dressing, and doing housework.

Core exercises can relieve low-back pain. And there's evidence they can improve physical functioning, mobility, and balance in older people. Strengthening your core may also improve your posture.

As for which core exercises are best, there's no definitive answer. One popular technique backed by research is Pilates, which combines aspects of gymnastics, martial arts, yoga, and dance. Other options include floor exercises such as crunches and planks; exercises on unstable surfaces like balls or balance boards; and exercises with weights. The *Fitter Faster* program includes a variety of effective core exercises that don't require any equipment.

CIRCUIT SHORTCUT

Conventional strength training typically involves doing several sets (a set is one round of reps) of an exercise and resting between sets for up to three minutes or longer, depending on how heavy the weights are. The rest periods can add up, making it hard to fit in a full-body workout if you're pressed for time.

Circuit training, in which you perform one set, move relatively quickly to the next exercise, and then repeat the circuit to do multiple sets, cuts the amount of time needed to do a full workout. Research suggests it can be just as beneficial as conventional strength training, if not more so.

For example, in a study of fit men in their 20s, researchers randomly assigned subjects to do either circuit training or conventional strength training. Each group did multiple sets. A third group served as a control. After eight weeks, both training groups had similar gains in strength and muscle mass, yet the circuit group had spent about 40 percent less time working out.

In a follow-up trial, the same researchers used a similar design to

Are home ab devices effective?

"Get ripped!" "Shed pounds and inches in just minutes a day." Go from "saggy flab to six-pack fab."

Those are among the come-ons for abdominal exercise contraptions that you've likely encountered on infomercials and in your spam folder. Typically they include before-and-after pictures of users, along with images of people with ripped abs who smile while they effortlessly work out.

To determine how well this equipment works, the American Council on Exercise commissioned a study to evaluate the effectiveness of eight popular devices along with seven conventional core exercises.

Placing electrodes on various core muscles, the researchers measured muscle activation as subjects performed each of the 15 exercises. While some of the devices equaled or even surpassed conventional exercises at working upper and lower abs, none was better than the traditional crunch.

Of course, the effectiveness of any exercise depends on whether you do it correctly. Though the researchers made certain that subjects used proper form, that doesn't always happen in the real world—whether you're doing crunches or using an ab contraption. A *Consumer Reports* study of one device, the Ab Coaster, found that fewer than half of the testers used it properly even with coaching from a fitness expert.

If an ab gadget motivates you to work out and you use it correctly, it may be worth the investment. But it won't necessarily produce better results than conventional ab exercises. And it alone definitely won't melt away belly fat and give you a six-pack. That requires reducing your overall body fat through diet along with cardio and strength training. Beware of any device manufacturer that claims otherwise.

study the effects in healthy men and women ages 55 to 75 with little or no experience working out. This time, subjects were followed for 12 weeks, and once again the circuit exercisers experienced improvements in strength and muscle mass comparable to those in the conventional training group. In addition, the two regimens resulted in similar increases in bone density.

What's more, circuit training led to greater decreases in body fat and improvements in markers of cardiovascular health than conventional strength training did. A likely reason is that limiting rest time keeps your heart rate up throughout the workout, especially if you're lifting heavier weights (as participants were in these studies).

Because of these advantages, we rely on circuit training in the *Fitter Faster* program. To keep the time commitment to a bare minimum, our plan requires just one set of each exercise, which studies show can be effective. However, on days you have more time, adding an extra set or two may yield even greater benefits.

Club Circuit

Some health clubs offer circuit-training programs, but often these regimens use relatively light weights, which can limit strength gains. As mentioned previously, our program varies the weights along with the number of reps.

Another difference is the types of weights used. Circuit training at health clubs typically involves exercise machines, while our program uses dumbbells along with body-weight exercises such as push-ups. That's due partly to convenience: You can do all our exercises at home and won't need to set foot in a gym if you don't want to.

Machines isolate specific muscles, which can be helpful for beginners learning proper form or for people recovering from injuries. But in real life, you rarely use your muscles in isolation. Dumbbells and other free weights better replicate reality because they force you to work additional muscles to keep your body stable and maintain your balance. This provides more effective "functional" training for everyday activities, whether you're carrying a bag of groceries or picking up an object off the floor.

An additional advantage of dumbbells is their versatility. They lend

If you do strength and cardio training in the same session, does the order matter?

Which type of exercise to do first has long been a matter of debate. Once I even witnessed a heated argument over the issue between two testosterone-laden weight lifters at my gym. (Fortunately, no punches were thrown.) The truth is that there's no one-size-fits-all answer. It depends on your exercise habits, priorities, and preferences.

Some research suggests that doing aerobic exercise first may reduce the effectiveness of strength training in the short run, perhaps by increasing muscle fatigue. But several studies tracking participants for longer periods have found that, over time, order doesn't matter. In one experiment, for example, researchers assigned physically active young men to do an aerobic workout (consisting of both steady-state and HIIT cycling) followed by strength training, or vice versa, two or three times a week. After six months, the two groups showed similar improvements in strength and aerobic fitness. Similarly, in a 12-week study involving older men, exercise order didn't affect strength gains.

What this research suggests is that if you double up on a regular basis, your body will adapt. If, however, you do so only occasionally, you may want to start with strength training if your main goal is to build muscle or strength. If you're training for a race, you may want to begin with aerobic exercise.

There's also the issue of which activity you enjoy more. As discussed in chapter 3, research suggests that starting with your favorite (or least objectionable) type of exercise may enhance the overall enjoyment of your workout. So if you prefer walking to weightlifting, begin with a walk.

The *Fitter Faster* workout program lets you avoid this dilemma by scheduling strength and aerobic exercise on different days. But if you're in the mood to do both, you'll need to experiment and see what order works better for you.

themselves to an endless array of exercises, which in various combinations can make up a full-body workout. Dumbbells even allow you to target disparate muscle groups, such as the shoulders and legs, with a single exercise. You'll find such movements, which are yet another way to increase the efficiency of your workouts, in the intermediate and advanced levels of our program.

A drawback of dumbbells is that you need to be extremely attentive to technique at all times. Using improper form—whether gripping the weights the wrong way, positioning your body incorrectly, straining your back, or swinging the dumbbells instead of raising and lowering them in a controlled manner—can cause injury and/or limit the effectiveness of your workouts. Dumbbell exercises usually take more time and effort than machines to master, but be patient. You'll get the hang of it!

ROOKIE ADVANTAGE

If you're new to strength training, you may see improvements after just one or two workouts. That's likely due mainly to adaptations by your nervous system in response to the new stimulus. In general, beginners experience strength gains more rapidly than others, with relatively large increases occurring after just a month or two in some people.

How much strength and size you gain, and how quickly, depends on a number of factors, including your age, gender, genetics, diet (more about that in chapter 8)—and, of course, effort. Keep in mind that not all muscle groups get bigger and stronger at the same rate. Though gains tend to slow as you do more strength training, they don't have to stop. As I've said, our program includes various features that help ensure that you'll continue progressing.

Still, it's important to keep your expectations realistic. You won't get ripped right away or perhaps ever. But if you do the workouts consistently, you will get stronger and eventually start seeing changes in your appearance. Take pride in these improvements. They're evidence of your hard work and can serve as a powerful incentive to keep pushing yourself.

Stretch Out

"You must be a runner," the instructor observed as I struggled through a yoga class. It was her kind way of telling me that my flexibility leaves a lot to be desired. But that wasn't news to me. I can barely touch my toes, and my Triangle Pose is not a pretty sight.

While genetics is partly to blame, it hasn't helped that I often give short shrift to stretching, which can improve flexibility. This is especially important as we age, when limited range of motion can make it harder to do everyday tasks, from getting dressed to reaching for objects on shelves. In addition, stretching may improve posture and balance. It helps prepare our bodies for exercise. Plus it feels good and can be relaxing.

Though stretching should be part of a comprehensive workout program, the wrong types of stretches before exercise can be ineffective and even counterproductive. The *Fitter Faster* program avoids this mistake by incorporating the right stretches before and after exercise and keeps the time required for them to a minimum.

Before I explain our approach, it's helpful to know how various forms of stretching differ and why much of what you've probably heard about stretching is misleading.

STRETCHING STYLES

Stretching comes in four basic varieties:

Static involves slowly stretching until you feel tightness and then holding the stretch. The most common type, it's relatively simple to do. Static stretches can be either active or passive: Active means that you use only the force of your own muscles (specifically, the ones opposite to the muscles being stretched) to do the stretch. Passive means that the stretch is performed with the help of an external force such as your hand, an elastic band, or a partner.

Ballistic entails bouncing to push beyond a muscle's normal range of motion. While it may be helpful for certain athletes, ballistic stretching can lead to injuries, so it's not recommended for most people.

Dynamic combines controlled movement with stretching. It works several muscles at the same time and is a good way to warm up before a workout. Examples of dynamic stretching include arm or leg swings.

PNF (short for proprioceptive neuromuscular facilitation) includes different techniques but generally involves contracting a muscle and then doing a static stretch of that muscle. Originally used for rehabilitation, PNF is typically done with a partner.

BENT TRUTH

Many of us learned in gym class or Little League that stretching before sports or exercise can prevent injury. Indeed, I remember doing toe touches and all kinds of other static stretches at the beginning of those unpleasant PE classes that I described in chapter 1. (Stretching was actually the least objectionable part.) The habit became so ingrained, as it has for many others, that I continued the practice for years before all my runs.

Alas, my efforts may have been in vain. In a study of 1,400 runners, researchers randomly assigned roughly half to do a series of static stretches before their runs. The rest didn't stretch. After three months, the injury rate among the stretchers was no lower than that of the non-stretchers.

The findings have been echoed by other trials involving runners, as well as military recruits and football players, which have also failed to show that static stretching prior to activity prevents injuries overall. It's possible that stretching may help reduce the chances of muscle strains from certain activities such as sprinting, but the evidence for this isn't ironclad.

Interestingly, in that study of 1,400 runners, participants who normally stretched before their runs but were assigned to the no-stretch group were nearly twice as likely to be injured as the non-stretchers assigned to the no-stretch group. What this suggests is that a sudden change in your training regimen may matter more than whether you stretch.

The evidence is even flimsier when it comes to another reason that many of us stretch: to prevent exercise-related soreness. A review of randomized studies found that stretching after exercise has virtually no effect on soreness a day or two later. On average, participants reported a reduction the next day of just one point on a 100-point scale. Stretching before exercise led to an even smaller decline in soreness. (For more on post-exercise soreness and the effectiveness of other methods in reducing it, see chapter 9.)

If stretching does decrease soreness, research suggests that people's beliefs and expectations may be responsible. In one of the reviewed studies, stretching was found to alleviate soreness in participants who strongly agreed that stretching is an important part of physical activity. But there was no such effect in subjects who strongly disagreed with that notion.

The Dark Side of Stretching

Unfortunately, the story of dashed hopes around stretching doesn't end there. Static stretching has actually been shown to do harm in certain cases.

A number of studies have found that static stretching before sports or exercise—especially when stretches are held for 60 seconds or longer—can impair performance. In a review of more than 100 studies,

Is foam rolling an effective alternative to stretching?

It's sometimes called the poor man's massage. But a growing number of not-so-poor athletes and others have embraced foam rolling, which involves using cylinders of various sizes, textures, and firmness levels to self-massage different areas of the body. The technique, known formally as self-myofascial release (SMR), can also be done with a roller massage bar (think rolling pin) or even a tennis ball.

Though the evidence is limited, the research we do have suggests that SMR may rival or even outshine stretching in certain ways. Two reviews of studies have found, for example, that SMR before or after exercise can increase range of motion. Combining SMR with static stretching may be more effective than either alone.

Further, SMR done after intense exercise and repeated for several days thereafter may reduce soreness. Unlike static and PNF stretching, SMR doesn't appear to impair athletic performance, and there's some evidence that the technique may even improve it.

Scientists aren't sure how SMR works, but a leading theory involves the fascia, which is web-like connective tissue that encases and connects muscles as well as bones, blood vessels, nerves, and internal organs. If adhesions form between layers of fascia—meaning they become stuck together—the result can be pain and reduced range of motion. SMR is thought to break up adhesions. It may also help by increasing blood flow.

SMR regimens and devices vary, and there's no consensus on which are best for whom. Studies do suggest, however, that rolling each area for 30 to 60 seconds may be optimal. If you try SMR, be sure to use proper technique, which includes: rolling slowly; maintaining good posture; not holding your breath; avoiding rolling your lower back and joints; and stopping if you feel sharp or severe pain.

researchers found that static stretching temporarily reduced muscular strength by as much as 10 percent or more, with an average of about 5 percent. Explosive muscular performance (which is required for activities such as sprinting and jumping) was decreased by an average of 2 percent. While these averages may not sound like much, being even a tad weaker and slower can make a difference, especially for athletes. Though there's less research on PNF stretching, it also appears to negatively affect performance.

Scientists have several theories as to why static and PNF stretching may be detrimental. One possibility is that a looser muscle acts like an overstretched slingshot, generating less force than one that's taut. Another hypothesis is that stretching "cold" muscles damages them. The nervous system may also play a role by trying to protect our muscles from harm when we stretch them—and, in the process, inhibiting them. Evidence for this effect includes the odd finding in some research that when a stretched limb loses strength, the same thing happens in the opposite limb—even though it wasn't stretched. Put another way, the left hand (or leg) may in fact know what the right one is doing.

WARM BODIES

Now that we've gotten through the shortcomings of stretching, let's turn to how it can be beneficial and how best to incorporate it. Before physical activity, you should warm up with a few minutes of low-intensity aerobic exercise such as relatively easy walking or jogging. The idea is to move enough to get your heart rate up, but not so much that you tire yourself out before you've even begun. Follow that with *dynamic* stretches such as arm circles, torso twists, and leg swings, all of which you'll find in the workouts in chapter 10.

Unlike static stretching, which as discussed can negatively affect your muscles prior to exercise, dynamic stretching primes them for action and may improve performance. In a study of young and middle-aged men, for example, vertical jump heights increased after dynamic stretching, while they declined after static stretching.

Similarly, a study involving female high school athletes found that they performed better on tests of balance, agility, and movement speed after dynamic stretching than after static stretching. And in a study of golfers, dynamic stretching led to greater clubhead speeds and ball speeds than static stretching. It also resulted in greater accuracy.

If you're playing golf or another sport, you should customize your stretching routine to involve the muscles that you'll be using. In that study of golfers, for example, participants targeted the legs, trunk, and shoulders with stretches such as butt kicks (kicking your heels to your derrière), walking lunges (taking giant steps out with your back knee bent and close to the ground), and torso twists combined with shoulder movements. After you stretch, do some activity-specific practice movements such as golf swings or tennis strokes.

If you participate in an activity such as gymnastics or dancing that requires a high level of flexibility and you want to do static stretching beforehand—or you're wedded to the practice and feel compelled to do it before your workout—hold each stretch for no longer than 30 seconds. Research shows that short static stretches are less likely to impair performance than longer ones. Precede the stretches with an aerobic warm-up and follow them with some dynamic stretches or activity-specific movements.

FLEX TIME

The best time to do static stretching or PNF is after physical activity, when your muscles are warm. Don't restrict your stretches to muscles that you've just taxed or ones that are tight. Instead, stretch muscles throughout your entire body, including those in the shoulders, chest, hips, back, and legs. Hold each stretch for 20 to 30 seconds while taking deep breaths. You should feel tightness or slight discomfort—but not pain, which can lead to injuries.

In the *Fitter Faster* plan, we've included static stretching exercises after workouts three days a week, which is consistent with recommendations by the American College of Sports Medicine. If you're able to stretch more often, research suggests that you may experience greater improvements in range of motion.

Of course, stretching exercises aren't the only way to increase flexibility. Yoga, Pilates, and tai chi can do the same while providing other health benefits as well. Though we haven't included these activities in

LEIGH
AGE 37
CAPE COD, MASSACHUSETTS

Leigh's job as a special education teacher was rewarding but also physically and emotionally demanding. "I found myself leaving work exhausted and sore," she says. Although accustomed to vigorous exercise from years of playing competitive sports, Leigh had never tried yoga. "After the first class, I was hooked," she says. The combination of movement, meditation, and breathing techniques helped Leigh cope with the challenges of her job and connect with her body in a way she had never experienced.

That connection made a difference in her other activities as well, including running the New York City marathon. "Yoga helped me with balance and range of motion during training," she says. "And it gave me a good sense of breath awareness and control." Leigh also turned to yoga during her pregnancy, when back pain became constant. "Breathing is such a big part of yoga, and I took those skills into the delivery room with me and definitely used them while I was recovering and nursing."

During her second pregnancy, three years later, Leigh once again found prenatal yoga classes to be invaluable. "I was so much busier because I was chasing a toddler," she says. "And my time on the mat became the only time I could truly be quiet and focused on my body and the new baby."

our plan, they can be a valuable part of a comprehensive exercise program. If you have the time and desire to incorporate any of them, by all means do so—perhaps on the "Your Choice" day of the *Fitter Faster* program. Just make certain you find a qualified instructor who can ensure that your technique is correct.

STRETCH OUT

FLEXIBILITY FACTORS

Studies have found that regular stretching can increase flexibility in as little as four weeks. But getting results requires commitment: You need to stretch at least three days a week, ideally every day. Though the *Fitter Faster* program calls for doing each stretch once, you should do two or three rounds if your goal is to increase flexibility and you have the time.

How flexible you are and how flexible you can become are also influenced by factors that you can't control, such as genetics and gender. (As anyone who has ever observed a co-ed yoga class can attest, women tend to be more flexible than men.) Injuries and certain conditions like arthritis can limit flexibility.

Age plays a role as well. Starting around age 30 or 40, flexibility continuously decreases, with men losing flexibility more quickly than women. This decline is thought to be due to decreases in muscle strength, cartilage resilience, and ligament elasticity that occur with age. The fact that many people become more sedentary as they age may also contribute, so it's possible that regular exercise can slow losses in flexibility. (Yet another reason to keep moving as we get older.)

Age-related changes in flexibility don't occur uniformly throughout the body. Research shows that the shoulders and trunk tend to lose flexibility more quickly than the elbows and knees, for example. At any age, you may be relatively flexible in one part of your body and have limited range of motion in another. Flexibility can also vary from one side to another; your right shoulder, for example, may have greater range of motion than your left shoulder, or vice versa.

As for how much flexibility is optimal, there's no definitive answer. We know that having poor range of motion can hamper athletic performance, increase the risk of injuries, and make tasks of daily living more difficult. It's also true that a high level of flexibility can be beneficial if you do activities such as gymnastics, swimming, or ballet. But this doesn't mean that we should all strive to become human pretzels.

Just as extreme inflexibility can lead to problems, so can extreme flexibility. People who are double-jointed—or have "joint hypermobility," as the condition is technically known—are more likely to experience pain and sports-related injuries. Interestingly, they're also at higher risk of anxiety disorders. (Why the two conditions are related is unknown.)

Does hot yoga increase flexibility more than conventional yoga?

It may seem like a circle of hell from a modern-day Dante's *Inferno* to some: throngs of sweaty bodies doing yoga poses for 90 minutes with the heat cranked up to over 100° Fahrenheit. But lots of people swear by hot yoga, or Bikram yoga, as the original version is known. In a survey of hot yoga practitioners, the most frequently reported benefit was increased flexibility, which was cited by nearly two thirds of respondents.

Though there's no definitive proof that hot yoga increases flexibility more than regular yoga, we do have circumstantial evidence. For example, a review of studies found that stretching muscles that are heated—whether with hot packs, ultrasound, or shortwave diathermy (which uses an electric current to produce heat)—improves range of motion more than stretching without heat. Also, the improvements appear to be longer lasting when muscles are heated.

Researchers aren't sure why heat increases flexibility, but they suspect it may be due to increased blood flow, relaxed muscles, or heat-induced changes in collagen and muscles.

Whatever the reasons, heat can also have a downside: It may make you more likely to overstretch, which can lead to injuries. That's one of the risks of hot yoga, along with dizziness, light-headedness, nausea, and dehydration. Of course you should stop and cool off if you experience any of these symptoms.

If hot yoga seems too daunting but you want to incorporate heat into your stretches, try doing them after applying hot packs to your muscles or while in a steamy shower (but make sure the shower has non-slip mats or treads so you won't fall). There's also the sauna or steam room—assuming you don't mind an audience.

Between the two extremes is a wide range of satisfactory flexibility levels. Being on the upper end of the range may impress your friends in yoga classes or games of Twister, but it won't necessarily confer any additional health benefits. Instead of worrying about how your flexibility stacks up against that of others, you should focus on what's right—and realistic—for yourself. Assess what your needs are and how stretching might address them. For example, maybe a certain part of your body is especially inflexible and holding you back in your workouts. Or perhaps you want to improve your flexibility in ways to help your tennis or golf game, or to get on the floor and play with your kids or grandkids.

Whatever the case, here are a few relatively simple tests you can use to assess your flexibility. While none is perfect, they can be useful for tracking your progress if you're trying to improve your range of motion. Do them after a warm-up or workout.

1. Sit and Reach

Developed in the 1950s, this classic test of flexibility in the hamstrings and lower back has several variations. Here's a DIY version from the YMCA that requires only a yardstick and masking tape.

Put the yardstick on the ground with a strip of tape across the 15-inch mark.

With your shoes off, sit on the floor with the yardstick between your legs and the 0-inch end closest to you.

Keep your legs straight and your feet about 12 inches apart. Sitting up straight, position your heels at the 14-inch mark.

Place one hand directly on top of the other and slowly reach forward as far as you can, without bouncing. Drop your head if it helps, and be sure to exhale as you stretch.

Note where the ends of your fingers reach on the yardstick. Repeat two more times, and record the farthest distance.

2. Zipper

This test of shoulder flexibility measures how closely you can bring your hands together behind your back. You need a tape measure or ruler and an assistant.

Stand and raise your right arm above your head. Bending your right elbow, reach behind your head with your palm touching your body. Reach as far down the middle of your back as you can, with your fingers pointed downward.

Place your left arm behind your back with your palm facing out and your fingers upward. Reach up as far as possible and try to touch your other hand.

Have someone measure the distance between the ends of your middle fingers. If they don't meet, record the length of the gap as a negative number. If they just touch, score that as a zero. If they overlap, record the length of the overlap as a positive number.

Do the test two more times and record your best reading. Then switch arms, putting your left hand behind your head, and repeat.

3. Sitting-Rising

This test, developed by a Brazilian doctor, has received attention as a tool to predict mortality risk in middle-aged and older people. But research suggests that it can also be an indicator of flexibility (as well as strength and balance) in people of all ages. No equipment is required, but you do need sufficient space to do the test and a surface that's not slippery.

Standing barefoot, try to sit on the floor with as little support as possible from your hands, legs, arms, or other body parts. Crossing your legs is fine.

From the seated position, try to stand up, again with as little support as possible.

Give yourself a score of 5 if you sat down with no support at all and 5 if you got up without support. For each support required, such as a hand, forearm, knee, side of a leg, or hand on a knee, subtract 1 point. Subtract a half point if you were wobbly sitting down or standing up.

Do the test twice and combine your best scores sitting and rising.

Get More Out of Exercise

What to Eat and How to Prevent Pain

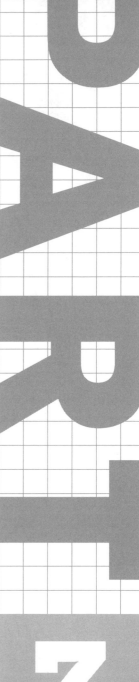

PART 3

Eat and Run

Hang around a health club long enough, and you'll likely hear chatter among gym rats about egg whites, steel-cut oats, protein powder, amino acid supplements, or other foods that are supposedly a must for enhancing workouts. This dietary advice might also include avoiding fruit, downing a gallon of distilled water, eating only at certain times, or consuming different foods on different days.

It can be tempting to believe that people with perfect physiques know what they're talking about, and indeed some of this "broscience" may work for some bodybuilders. But much of it is folklore that in any case isn't even relevant to the needs of most people. What the skinny guys in glasses—that is, the researchers conducting real science—tell us is that unless you're a competitive athlete, eating for exercise doesn't require special foods or complicated regimens. The *Fitter Faster* plan involves simply eating a healthful diet, with special attention to protein, carbohydrates, and hydration.

PICK YOUR PROTEIN

When you eat protein, it's broken down into amino acids, which the body uses for a number of things, including forming new protein in muscle. That's important because muscle protein is constantly being made and degraded by our bodies. As discussed in chapter 6, resistance training causes injury to muscle cells, to which our bodies respond by forming new muscle protein. If levels of amino acids are sufficient, the amount of muscle protein formed exceeds the amount broken down, and the result is an increase in muscle size and strength.

So how much protein is sufficient to maintain or increase muscle? The Recommended Dietary Allowance (RDA) for protein is .36 grams of protein per pound of body weight a day—a number that many experts believe is too low. By contrast, some bodybuilders and other athletes take in three times that amount or more. While such levels are not thought to cause harm (unless you have kidney disease), they exceed what most of us need.

The Goldilocks amount for most of us appears to be around .5 grams per pound, which makes it easy to calculate. Just cut your weight in half—so someone who weighs 140 pounds should get 70 grams of protein a day; a person who tips the scales at 200 needs 100 grams.

Competitive athletes who participate in power sports or endurance competitions may require more—up to around .9 grams per pound. The same goes for people doing resistance training who are trying to maximize gains in strength or lean body mass. And those who exercise vigorously while on a low-calorie diet, which can lead to muscle loss, may benefit from extra protein.

Studies have found that eating 20 or 30 grams of protein at a time is generally optimal for muscle-protein formation and that larger doses aren't any more effective. As for timing, it's best to get protein throughout the day rather than consuming the bulk of it at dinner, as many people do. While it's conventional wisdom in the athletic world that downing protein within an hour or so after strength training is necessary to maximize gains, the research on this is mixed. The science is even less conclusive on whether consuming protein after aerobic exercise is beneficial.

A normal diet can supply enough protein for most people. The best sources are chicken or turkey breast, beef, and pork, which typically have at least 30 grams per four-ounce serving. Fish and shellfish such as salmon, tuna, and shrimp rank up there as well. Many dairy products, especially Greek yogurt and cottage cheese, are also good sources. Egg whites, despite their exalted reputation among many body builders, deliver only about 3.5 grams of protein each. Whole eggs have more—

around 6 grams—and they can be part of a healthful diet. Research shows that eating up to seven a week doesn't raise blood cholesterol levels or increase the risk of heart disease for most people.

Choosing from just the above foods, someone who weighed 175 pounds and ate two scrambled eggs for breakfast (12 grams), a salad topped with chicken breast for lunch (30 grams), a 6-ounce Greek yogurt for a snack (17 grams), and a medium-sized salmon fillet for dinner (30 grams) would meet his or her daily requirement of 88 grams of protein.

And that doesn't even include the many plant sources of protein. Topping the list of these are tofu, soy nuts, and veggie burgers. Soymilk, beans, and seeds are also decent sources. Ditto for peanut butter and nuts, though milks made from almonds and cashews contain very little protein. You also get protein from grains such as oats, wheat, rice, and quinoa.

A downside of plant proteins is that most are "incomplete," meaning that they don't contain all of the nine amino acids that we need from food to form muscle protein. Because our bodies can't manufacture these "essential" amino acids, as they're called, we have to rely on our diets for them. (The body does make another 11 amino acids.) Only a few plant proteins, such as soy and quinoa, include all the essential amino acids in sufficient amounts. In contrast, all animal proteins, such as poultry, meat, fish, dairy products, and eggs, are "complete," which means they contain all the amino acids that we require.

If you're a vegetarian, it can be harder to get enough of the essential amino acids—and enough protein generally—but it's certainly doable if you choose your foods carefully. If you're a vegan or on a low-calorie diet, protein supplements may be necessary.

PLAY YOUR CARBS RIGHT

When we eat carbohydrates, our bodies convert them to glucose. Most of this is then stored as glycogen in the muscles and liver. During exercise, our muscles break down the glycogen and use it for energy.

Though you may have heard about marathon runners or other athletes "carbo-loading" before an event, this isn't necessary for recreational athletes, and it may weigh you down by adding water weight. A

Which type of protein supplement is best?

Most protein powders, drinks, and bars are made from whey, casein, or soy protein, or some combination of these. Studies comparing these forms tend to be small with conflicting results, and much of the research is funded by vested interests such as the dairy industry. All this makes definitive answers hard to come by, but here are some basics to keep in mind.

Whey, which is a byproduct of cheese production, is a complete protein. It's higher than any other protein in leucine, an amino acid that's especially important for the formation of muscle protein. As a result, it enjoys a reputation as the ideal protein source. However, it may cause gastrointestinal upset in people who are lactose-intolerant. To avoid this, choose products with whey isolate (as opposed to whey concentrate), which typically has very little lactose.

Like whey, casein is a milk protein that's complete. But it's absorbed more slowly than whey. As a result, it may be a good option before bed so the body can be supplied with protein throughout the night. It may also help you feel full longer during the daytime.

Soy is a complete protein as well, which makes it an especially good option for vegans. Despite rumors that it has feminizing effects in men such as suppressing testosterone, increasing estrogen, or producing man-boobs, the research as a whole has failed to prove any of this. However, soy may adversely affect thyroid levels in certain people, especially those who have, or are predisposed to, thyroid disease.

If you don't want milk-based or soy protein, another option is egg protein. Derived from egg whites, it's complete. You can also find products containing other plant sources such as peas, rice, or hemp. But because they're less complete than other types, it's probably best to combine plant proteins rather than relying on just one.

normal diet that includes sources of carbohydrates such as fruits, veggies, beans, cereal, bread, pasta, rice, and sweets typically results in sufficient glycogen levels to fuel muscles for up to about 90 minutes of exercise.

For vigorous activities lasting longer than that, such as marathons or triathlons, consuming carbs one to four hours beforehand has been shown to increase endurance. Foods low in fat and fiber are generally best because they're less likely to cause gastrointestinal upset. If you want some fuel right before exercise—when you work out first thing in the morning, for example—a light, easily digestible snack such as a banana, oatmeal, or a piece of whole-grain toast with jam can do the trick.

You don't need carbohydrates (or any other food) during your activity unless it's one that's prolonged and intense, such as a marathon. In that case, a sports drink or gel is often the best option.

As for what to eat immediately afterward, carbs may help endurance athletes, especially if they have another training session later in the day. Some research suggests that chocolate milk is an ideal recovery food for such athletes because its combination of sugar and protein (a 4-to-1 ratio of carbs to protein) appears to be optimal for rapidly replenishing glycogen in muscles.

But before you reach for the Hershey's syrup, keep in mind that chocolate milk or any other food is unnecessary after *Fitter Faster* workouts or other typical exercise. If you're hungry and want to refuel, try a light carb-and-protein snack such as plain yogurt and fruit. Just be sure to keep an eye on calories. If you're watching your weight, adding calories after your workouts—without reducing them sufficiently elsewhere in your diet—could undermine your efforts.

DRINK, BUT NOT TO EXCESS

We've all heard the advice that everyone needs eight glasses of water a day, even if we're not thirsty. Likewise, conventional wisdom (much of it influenced by makers of sports beverages such as Gatorade) has it that you should "stay ahead of your thirst" before, during, and after exercise to avoid dehydration, which impairs performance and causes harm.

It turns out that such notions may be all wet. Research shows that most people typically get enough water through foods (which supply

20 percent of our water) and beverages (including coffee, tea, soda, juice, and milk), and that thirst is a reliable indicator of when we need more fluid, even during exercise.

A review of studies involving competitive cyclists has found that mild dehydration does not impair exercise performance. What's more, drinking only when thirsty results in better performance than does chugging constantly. Other research shows that contrary to popular belief and the advice on many websites, dehydration is not generally a cause of exercise-related muscle cramps or heat illness.

Though you want to make sure to consume enough water, especially if you're older or exercising in the heat, a bigger problem than dehydration may be drinking *too much* during exercise, according to a report authored by a panel of 17 experts. If you take in so much fluid that your body can't get rid of the excess through sweating or urination, sodium levels can become dangerously low. The resulting condition, known as hyponatremia or water intoxication, can cause headaches, vomiting, confusion, seizures, and, in some cases, death.

Previously, hyponatremia occurred mainly in slower marathon runners, but the report says it's now also showing up among people engaged in activities such as hiking, half-marathons, hot yoga, military exercises, and football at the high school, college, and professional levels. To prevent the condition and stay hydrated, the best strategy "before, during, and immediately following exercise," the report concludes, "is to drink palatable fluids when thirsty."

If for you "palatable fluids" include plain water, that's your best bet. If not, you can find flavored waters or use flavor drops or powders. One possible downside of these products is that they often contain artificial sweeteners or other additives. If you're looking for something more natural, add a splash of juice, some slices of fruit, or sprigs of herb.

Sports beverages, which contain fluids, carbohydrates, and minerals known as electrolytes, can be useful for athletes engaged in vigorous exercise for more than an hour, especially in hot weather. But for most of us, they offer no benefits over water while providing extra calories and sugar that we don't need.

Like sports beverages, some bottled waters contain added sodium along with other electrolytes. For people who do strenuous exercise for more than an hour or sweat very heavily, electrolytes—which replace salts lost through sweat—may help head off dehydration. But in many cases, the levels of electrolytes in enhanced waters are too low to help, so food or a sports beverage may be a better source.

Coconut water, which is also touted as an alternative to sports drinks, is high in the electrolyte potassium. But coconut water typically contains less sodium than sports beverages, a feature that makes it less effective for those doing prolonged, vigorous exercise. While some people prefer coconut water's taste to that of regular water, coconut water also has more calories.

Despite the hype surrounding other special waters, such as those that are alkaline, distilled, oxygenated, or vitamin-enhanced, there's little evidence that they're more beneficial than regular water when it comes to hydration, athletic performance, recovery, or general health.

BE SELECTIVE WITH SUPPLEMENTS

Whether you're a competitive athlete or an occasional exerciser, it can be hard to resist the allure of pills and powders that promise to let you go faster, lift more weight, or feel less fatigued. You can find a dizzying array of fitness supplements online, at gyms, or on the shelves of supplement shops, health-food stores, pharmacies, and supermarkets.

Most of these products haven't been proven to work, some could be harmful, and none are necessary for exercise. But if you're looking for a competitive edge, there are a few standouts that have proven benefits and, based on what's currently known, appear to be relatively safe. Others have more limited science behind them but enough to suggest that they may be effective for at least some people. Here's the lowdown on a few popular supplements.

Does dark urine mean you're dehydrated?

Check the color of your pee: You've probably encountered this advice on how to tell whether you're adequately hydrated. We often hear that urine ideally should be pale yellow and that the darker it is, the more we're dehydrated.

It turns out that the science behind such guidance isn't so clear. In a review of the evidence, researchers peed all over the notion that urine color is an accurate marker of hydration. Part of the problem is that some foods (such as beets and carrots) can affect the color of urine, as can certain vitamins. Ditto for some medications and dietary supplements. What's more, striving for pale pee could prompt some people to drink too much, overhydrate themselves, and develop water intoxication.

If you're concerned that your workout routine is leaving you dehydrated, try weighing yourself, without clothes, before and after exercise. If you lose a few pounds, you're likely okay. If you lose more than that, you may want to increase your fluid intake. If, on the other hand, you gain weight, you may be drinking too much.

Creatine: *Standout*

Creatine, an amino acid produced in the body and stored mainly in muscle, helps provide quick energy to muscles when we need it. Overall, research shows that when combined with resistance training, creatine can increase muscle mass and strength in both young adults and older people more than resistance training alone. It may also help improve performance at high-intensity exercises lasting less than 30 seconds.

Dietary sources include meat, poultry, and fish, a fact that may explain why vegetarians (who don't consume these foods) especially appear to benefit from creatine supplements. You can find various forms of creatine on shelves, but the most widely studied is creatine monohydrate. It's fine to take the supplement either before or after a workout, and research suggests that combining it with carbohydrate, protein, or both increases creatine's effectiveness. To maximize the amount of creatine in muscle tissue, many people start with a "loading" dose of around 20 grams per day for the first week or so and then take 3 to 5 grams a day after that.

These amounts are thought to be safe for most people, though creatine can cause stomach cramps and diarrhea as well as dehydration, which is why it's wise to drink lots of water when taking the supplement. People with kidney problems should avoid creatine. Any long-term risks are unknown because such research hasn't been conducted.

Caffeine: *Standout*

A large body of research shows that caffeine can improve performance in endurance activities like running or cycling. In addition, it may also provide a boost for high-intensity exercises such as jumping, sprinting, and weightlifting.

Scientists aren't exactly sure why caffeine works. One longstanding theory, which some researchers now dispute, is that caffeine causes fats to be used for energy. This conserves glycogen for later use during exercise, which delays fatigue. Caffeine also affects the brain, boosting alertness and mood, and reducing perceived effort. People who aren't regular users appear to benefit most.

The effects of caffeine peak about an hour after it's ingested. The optimal dose for athletes appears to be 3 to 6 milligrams per kilogram of body weight. For someone who weighs 150 pounds (70 kilograms), that translates to roughly 200 to 400 milligrams of caffeine—the amount in several cups of coffee.

Speaking of coffee, there's some evidence that it can provide an exercise boost, but overall the research is mixed. The same goes for another common caffeine source, energy drinks and shots, with some studies showing that they improve performance and others finding that they don't. One possible reason for the conflicting results is that coffee and energy drinks also contain other compounds, which may blunt the effects of caffeine.

In addition, similar products can vary in the amount of caffeine they contain. Because of that—and the fact that caffeine levels aren't always listed on foods, drinks, or energy shots—it can be tough to figure out how much you're getting from these products. We do know that sodas and most teas generally contain too little caffeine to be effective unless you drink very large amounts.

While caffeine is available in a wide array of products from gels to chewing gums, most studies have used pure caffeine in the form of capsules. That's generally a good way to get caffeine, as long as you don't exceed the recommended amount. However, steer clear of powders, which have been linked to the deaths of people who accidentally overdosed. A single teaspoon contains the amount of caffeine in 28 cups of coffee, and accurately measuring the powder with kitchen utensils can be tricky.

You don't need to ingest massive amounts of caffeine, in whatever form, to experience side effects, which can include insomnia, jitteriness, and stomach upset. In addition, caffeine can increase heart rate and decrease blood flow to the heart during exercise, which for some people may impair athletic performance rather than improve it.

Beta Alanine: *Maybe*

Beta alanine is an amino acid produced in the body. Though results have been mixed, overall the evidence suggests that beta alanine supplements may improve performance and reduce fatigue, especially during high-intensity bursts of activity lasting one to four minutes. And it's not just young athletes who seem to benefit. In several trials involving healthy people in their 70s, 80s, and even 90s, subjects showed improvements on exercise tests such as cycling and treadmill-walking after taking beta alanine.

Beta alanine is thought to work by increasing levels of a compound in muscles called carnosine, which may help reduce exercise-related fatigue by decreasing acidity in muscles. Research shows that a "loading" dose of 4 to 6 grams of beta alanine a day for a month or longer can boost carnosine by as much as 80 percent. But taking this much beta alanine at once can cause a tingling sensation, so the dose needs to be split into smaller amounts. This side effect can also be minimized with a slow-release version of the supplement.

The optimal dose for ongoing use of beta alanine hasn't been firmly established. Nor do scientists know whether there are any long-term side effects.

Branched-Chain Amino Acids: *Maybe*

The branched-chain amino acids (BCAA), so named because of their chemical structure, include isoleucine, leucine, and valine. All are essential, meaning that the body can't produce them. As mentioned previously, leucine appears to be especially important for muscle-protein formation.

A handful of studies show that taking BCAA supplements may decrease muscle soreness after exercise. (For more on preventing soreness, see chapter 9.) BCAAs haven't been shown to improve athletic performance, but feeling less sore may make exercise more doable.

Studies have used different regimens and doses of BCAAs (ranging from 2 to 20 grams), so the optimal timing and amount are unclear.

The jury is also still out on whether BCAA supplements provide benefits beyond those from a diet rich in BCAA-rich foods such as dairy, eggs, meat, chicken, and fish. People who avoid these foods, or who are on a low-calorie diet, may get a bigger boost from BCAA supplements. Aside from possibly interfering with certain medications for diabetes and other conditions, BCAA supplements are thought to be safe.

Testosterone Boosters: *Forget It*

Bodybuilding supplements claiming to increase testosterone levels and muscle strength, which often contain ingredients such as tribulus terrestris, D-aspartic acid (DAA), or ZMA, have little science to support their use. What's worse, some products such as those that purport to be "natural" versions of anabolic steroids have been found to illegally contain synthetic steroids, which are considered drugs. The Food and Drug Administration (FDA) has received reports of serious side effects such as

Should I buy this supplement?

If you're shopping for a dietary supplement for fitness (or any other purpose), "buyer beware" are the operative words. Manufacturers aren't required to demonstrate that supplements are safe or effective before selling them. What's more, there's no guarantee that the products actually contain what's listed on labels, and the levels of some ingredients, especially in multi-ingredient supplements, may be too low to be effective.

Following these tips can help you be a savvier supplement shopper.

- Ignore claims such as "clinically proven" or "clinically tested," which are basically meaningless. Instead, check out the research for yourself by going to Google Scholar or PubMed.gov. Look for independent studies testing that type of supplement in people—not in animals or test tubes.
- Beware of supplements containing a "proprietary blend" of ingredients. This can include a hodgepodge of things that you don't want and insufficient amounts of what you do want. Don't take more than the recommended amount.
- See if the product has been tested by Consumerlab.com or Labdoor.com. Both of these independent organizations analyze dietary supplements to see whether they contain what's listed on the label as well as any impurities or potentially harmful ingredients.
- Don't be swayed by claims that a supplement or its ingredients are "natural." Just because something is natural doesn't necessarily mean it's safe.

liver failure, stroke, and kidney failure linked to some of these supplements. That may be just the tip of the iceberg since there's very limited research on their ingredients and how they affect the body.

Antioxidants: *Forget It*

Exercise boosts the production of free radicals, which can damage cells. Antioxidants neutralize free radicals, so antioxidant supplements such as vitamins C and E are touted as a way for athletes to prevent this damage and improve performance.

But overall, research has failed to show that antioxidant supplements live up to their billing. And a number of studies suggest that they may even block some of the benefits of exercise, including increases in strength, lean body mass, and insulin sensitivity, by inhibiting the body's natural response to free radicals. As one team of researchers put it, the supplements are "at the least, useless."

That doesn't mean, however, that a diet high in antioxidants is useless. Research shows that antioxidant-rich foods like blueberries, oranges, almonds, and sweet potatoes are beneficial for overall health.

EIGHT EATING RULES

Whatever benefits that pills, powders, or sports drinks may provide to some athletes, they pale in comparison to those of a proper diet. And no product can make up for poor eating. As for the optimal diet for exercise, there's no one-size-fits-all regimen. A young man wanting to put on muscle, for example, requires a different diet than a middle-aged woman seeking to lose weight. Still, some general principles of healthful eating apply to everyone following the *Fitter Faster* program:

1. Include protein at every meal from sources such as poultry, fish, eggs, dairy, beans, nuts, or tofu. Go easy on red and processed meats. If you're a vegetarian, make sure you eat a variety of plant proteins, since most aren't complete.

115

2. Go for complex carbohydrates, which include whole grains, beans, and fruit. Eat plenty of vegetables, *and* keep refined carbs such as white bread, chips, cookies, candies, and other sugary foods to a minimum.

3. Incorporate "good" fats such as olive oil, fatty fish, avocado, nuts, and seeds. Remember that low-fat doesn't necessarily equal healthful. Avoid fried foods.

4. When it comes to beverages, stick mainly with water. Minimize your intake of soda, including diet soda, which may stimulate appetite. Keep in mind that fruit juice can have as much sugar as soda, so consume it sparingly. And drink alcohol in moderation—meaning at most one drink a day for women and two for men.

5. Forget about fad diets. Eating plans that require you to do things such as consuming (or shunning) specific foods, eating different foods on different days, or confining your eating to certain hours are too restrictive and complicated to follow for very long. Over the long run, they don't work for weight loss, nor have they been proven to enhance exercise performance.

6. Check out the ingredient list on packaged foods. If it includes a string of unpronounceable words, consider it a red flag. Generally, a shorter list means the food is less processed.

7. Ignore health-related marketing claims on packages. Just because a food or drink is labeled with terms such as "organic," "natural," "multigrain," "gluten-free," or "vitamin-fortified" doesn't necessarily mean it's healthful. When foods are marketed with this type of "health halo," people are more likely to overeat them, according to research. The same is true for snacks like energy bars that are branded as "fitness" foods.

8. If you do buy energy bars, read labels carefully. Some are relatively high in calories and have as much sugar as candy. In some cases, products are sweetened with sugar substitutes known as sugar alcohols (typically identifiable with words ending in -*ol* on the ingredient list), which can cause gas, bloating, and diarrhea. Also, check to see whether there are added vitamins, minerals, or caffeine, which you may not want or need.

CATHERINE

AGE 24

CAPE TOWN, SOUTH AFRICA

Participating in competitive equestrian events required Catherine to stay in excellent shape. She did so by working out four or five times a week, sometimes for more than three hours at a time. Though she'd gotten a clean bill of health from her doctor and wasn't overweight, this superfit athlete often lacked energy and didn't feel very good. She napped frequently and typically hit the snooze button several times before getting out of bed. Catherine's instincts told her that something was amiss. "I knew this wasn't how I was supposed to feel, since I was young and healthy," she recalls. "I figured maybe it was from stress or just too much exercise."

Encouragement from a family member prompted Catherine to try changing her diet. She started by replacing her morning sugary cereal with a protein shake and fruit. For lunch, she bypassed pizza or deli sandwiches for salads with chicken. She felt different almost immediately. "I could tell right away I had more energy," Catherine says. "And I stopped hitting the snooze button!"

Her newfound energy led Catherine to research more ways to change her eating habits. "I started eating several small meals a day instead of just two big ones, and I stopped eating so late at night," she says. Catherine hadn't set out to lose weight, but her body did change: "My muscles became more pronounced, especially in my arms and back, and my pants were looser."

No longer a competitive athlete, Catherine now stays in shape by working out two or three times a week, walking her dog, and mountain biking. She doesn't deny herself the occasional sugar or starch, but she knows that eating processed foods makes her feel sluggish. "People ask me how long I'm going to keep this up, and I laugh," she says. "I remember how it felt to be tired all the time. Why would I ever want to feel that way again?"

Feel No (Bad) Pain

I have a confession: I don't mind exercise-related pain. In fact, I welcome it. Now, before you conclude that I'm a masochist, let me explain: The type of pain I'm talking about is soreness that comes after exercise and may last for a few days before going away. Known as delayed onset muscle soreness, or DOMS for short, it's a sign that your workout is making you stronger. I consider it "good" pain. What I definitely *don't* like or welcome is "bad" pain, which typically happens during exercise and gets worse afterward. It's a sign that you have an injury.

While you probably don't share my odd affinity for DOMS, chances are that you've experienced this type of soreness at some point or will experience it, especially if you're new to exercise. DOMS typically begins 12 to 24 hours after a workout and reaches its peak on the second or third day following exercise. Any type of activity can cause this type of soreness, especially if the exercise is strenuous or something to which your body isn't accustomed. However, DOMS is most likely to occur after muscle-lengthening (or eccentric) movements such as lowering a dumbbell or running downhill.

For nearly a century, DOMS was widely attributed to the buildup of lactic acid in muscles. Today, lactic acid retains its reputation among some in the fitness world as a pain-causing waste product. But, science has shown that to be a bum rap. Our muscles break down glucose into lactic acid (technically, lactate), which is used as fuel. Lactate is removed from muscle within a few hours after exercise, so lactic acid can't explain soreness that occurs a day or two later.

Instead, researchers now believe that the discomfort is due to the process by which the body repairs micro-tears in muscle caused by exercise. (For more on this, see pages 79–80.) Soreness isn't the only symptom; swelling, stiffness, tenderness, and a reduction in strength and range of motion can also occur. These usually go away within several days. When you do the same activity again, your DOMS will likely be milder—or won't occur at all. And you'll be stronger.

However, soreness isn't required for strength gains. You can have an effective workout without DOMS, so don't worry that you're wasting your time if you don't feel sore. No pain doesn't necessarily mean no gain.

It's generally fine to exercise with DOMS, though you may need to dial back the intensity or focus on areas not affected—for example, working out your upper body if your legs are sore. Taking a day off to rest is okay, but don't use DOMS as an excuse for an extended (or permanent) break from exercise.

In fact, physical activity may decrease your soreness, at least while you're doing the activity. BCAA supplements and compression clothing may have an effect as well. (See pages 50–51 and 113.) However, as discussed in chapter 7, stretching doesn't appear to help. Other methods promoted for DOMS relief include heat and cold, massage, painkillers, and tart cherry juice, some of which have more promise than others.

Fire and Ice

Though heat and cold have been used for centuries to relieve pain, the evidence for their effectiveness at reducing DOMS is mixed. One reason is that different studies have applied heat or cold in different ways, at different temperatures, for different lengths of time.

Methods of delivering heat include hot packs, ultrasound, saunas, and warm water, which vary in their ability to penetrate beneath the skin into deep tissue. Cold therapy can come in the form of cold packs, ice massage, or ice baths.

In a review of 17 trials of ice-bath treatments, which are often used by athletes, researchers concluded that the technique may reduce soreness after exercise. But sitting in a tub of water chilled to 50-something degrees Fahrenheit—ideally for 10 to 15 minutes, according to research—isn't exactly pleasant.

A relatively new method is whole-body cryotherapy (WBC), in which you sit or stand for two to four minutes in a special chamber where the temperature is as low as -300°F. (No, that's not a typo.) A review of four studies found that there's insufficient evidence to tell whether WBC reduces DOMS. And potential risks, which include frostbite, oxygen deficiency, and asphyxiation, have yet to be studied.

The conventional wisdom, with little direct evidence to support it, has been that cold is superior to heat in reducing DOMS. To test this idea, researchers did a randomized, head-to-head comparison. One hundred young adults performed squats for 15 minutes and then received one of four therapies: 1) cold wraps immediately after exercise; 2) cold wraps 24 hours after exercise; 3) heat wraps immediately after exercise; 4) heat wraps 24 hours after exercise. A fifth group, which served as a control, received no treatment.

Cold wraps were placed on both legs for 20 minutes. Heat wraps were left on subjects' legs for eight hours to give adequate time for the heat to penetrate deeply into muscle. (The temperature—about 104°F—was low enough so as not to burn the skin.) The verdict: Both heat and cold therapy reduced soreness, but cold—whether applied immediately after exercise or 24 hours later—was superior to heat.

Though scientists aren't sure exactly why cold or heat might reduce DOMS, it is known that the two have opposite physiological effects: Cold constricts blood vessels and reduces blood flow, while heat dilates vessels and increases flow. Based on this, some athletes alternate between cold and heat, which they claim creates a "pumping action" of constriction and dilation that removes waste products from muscles and brings in fresh blood. Known as contrast therapy, this approach typically involves one or two minutes in a cold bath followed by a warm bath, and then repeating the sequence multiple times.

Pooling data from 13 studies, researchers found that contrast therapy decreases post-exercise soreness more than resting does. But it doesn't appear to offer any advantages over cold water alone. While it's possible that longer times in the water might yield different results, all the tub-hopping probably isn't worth the effort.

Rubbing Elbows (and Other Body Parts)

Getting a massage is certainly more enjoyable than sitting in a cold bath, and research suggests it may reduce DOMS, at least temporarily. In a review of nine studies on massage, six of them found that it alleviated soreness. The rub, however, is that the benefit generally occurred only in the early stages of DOMS, at 24 hours post-exercise. At 48 and 72 hours after exercise, there was less evidence that massage helped.

Though researchers aren't sure why massage reduces pain, possible explanations include its effects on inflammation, stress hormones, or the nervous system. Another theory is that massage increases blood flow to muscles, though some studies refute this idea and even show that massage may have the opposite effect. Perhaps the most common explanation is that it works by removing lactic acid. But, as previously mentioned, lactic acid isn't a cause of DOMS.

Because studies have used different massage techniques, it's unclear which methods are most effective. There's also uncertainty about timing and duration, though in most of the studies that showed a benefit, massages were done two or three hours after exercise and lasted 20 to 30 minutes.

One possible downside of massage is the cost. But, as discussed in chapter 7, self-massage performed with a foam roller may be a relatively inexpensive alternative—assuming you don't go wild on candles and incense.

Bitter Pill

Many athletes routinely take nonsteroidal anti-inflammatory drugs (NSAIDs), a class of painkillers that includes ibuprofen (Advil, Motrin) and naproxen (Aleve), as a preventive measure to head off pain during competition and DOMS afterward. Of the possible ways to reduce soreness, taking pills is certainly the simplest. But the truth about their effects is complicated.

NSAIDs, which are effective for relieving various types of pain, work by reducing inflammation. Since DOMS involves inflammation, it stands to reason that the medications would help alleviate post-exercise soreness. But research by and large has failed to prove that they do. For example, in a study of participants in the Western States Endurance Run, an arduous 100-mile race, 29 runners took ibuprofen on the day before and during the race, while 25 didn't take the drug or other medications. The ibuprofen users experienced just as much soreness afterward as the non-users.

What's more, when researchers analyzed blood samples from the racers, they found signs of adverse effects in those who had used ibuprofen. The most worrisome was mild endotoxemia, a condition in which intestinal bacteria get into the bloodstream. Scientists think this occurs because exercise and ibuprofen, when combined, gang up on the gastrointestinal system. Strenuous exercise can cause short-term injury to the lining of the small intestine, and taking ibuprofen—which itself can lead to gastrointestinal damage—may aggravate the problem, according to research. The result is increased intestinal permeability, which may allow bacteria to leak out of the gut.

Another potential concern is that ibuprofen and other NSAIDs may limit gains from resistance training. Studies in rodents support this idea, and there's a biological basis for it: NSAIDs suppress the production of substances known as prostaglandins, which are involved in the body's response to exercise-related muscle damage and the formation of muscle protein.

But several studies in humans have shown that up to 1,200 milligrams a day of ibuprofen (the amount you typically get in six over-the-counter pills) has no detrimental effects on muscle growth or strength gains, at least in the short run. It's still unknown, however, whether regular, long-term use of ibuprofen or higher doses can impede progress.

The take-home message is that the possible downsides of using NSAIDs to reduce DOMS on a regular basis likely outweigh any benefits. As for acetaminophen (Tylenol), there's no evidence that it causes gastrointestinal damage or interferes with resistance training. But unfortunately there's also little evidence that it reduces DOMS.

FEEL NO (BAD) PAIN

Bowls of Cherries

It used to be that cherries were best known as pie filler. Today they have a reputation as a "superfood" with a number of health benefits, one of which is that cherry juice supposedly reduces DOMS. Though the research is preliminary, there is some evidence to support the idea.

For example, in a small, randomized study, male college students drank either tart cherry juice or a placebo beverage for four days, did bicep curls to induce DOMS, and then drank their assigned beverage for another four days. Those consuming the cherry juice reported less soreness than the non-juice-drinkers, and their pain peaked and declined more rapidly. The research was funded by a cherry-juice manufacturer.

In a study not funded by industry, semi-professional soccer players consumed tart cherry concentrate (which was mixed with water) or a placebo for eight days. On day five, they ran sprint intervals. Post-exercise soreness was lower in those who had gotten the tart cherry concentrate.

But stopping there would amount to cherry-picking studies. Other research involving marathon runners and cyclists has found no reductions in DOMS among subjects consuming tart cherry juice or concentrate. Researchers theorize that differences in the types of exercise—and specifically whether they involve eccentric muscle action—may help explain the conflicting results.

As for how tart cherries might alleviate pain, they're rich in substances known as anthocyanins, which are known to act like NSAIDs and reduce inflammation. And research in rats has found tart cherry anthocyanins to have pain-reducing effects similar to those of NSAIDs.

Though the optimal dose is unknown, subjects in studies consumed the equivalent of about 100 cherries per day, which you can typically get in two cups of tart cherry juice or a smaller amount of concentrate. If you follow the regimen for multiple days, as was done in research, the extra calories and sugar can quickly add up. That may be a price for pain relief that you don't want to pay.

Does cupping reduce pain?

Though cupping has been around since ancient times, many people first learned about the Chinese healing practice when swimmer Michael Phelps used it during the 2016 Olympics.

A version known as "dry" cupping involves placing cups over the skin and using either a pump or heat to create vacuum pressure. This causes capillaries to rupture, resulting in purple circles that look like hickeys. In "wet" cupping, the skin is punctured before the cups are placed on it.

Phelps and other athletes claim that cupping reduces soreness and speeds healing, but the science behind this is skimpy. While some studies suggest that the practice may provide short-term relief for certain types of acute and chronic pain, reviews of the research have found that most of the studies are of poor quality, making it hard to draw any conclusions. What's more, none of the studies has focused specifically on exercise-related muscle pain.

Scientists suspect that cupping's effect on pain, if there is one, may be due to increased blood flow. It's also possible that any apparent benefits are in people's minds: Those who report relief *think* it makes them feel better.

In any event, there appear to be no major side effects, especially from dry cupping. So if you want to sport purple circles like Michael Phelps, go for it. Just don't expect it to make you an Olympic swimmer.

The takeaway is that while some methods touted for reducing soreness may provide a bit of relief, all have shortcomings and none is guaranteed to keep DOMS at bay. With or without these remedies, you'll likely experience some degree of soreness after workouts in the *Fitter Faster* program, especially if you're not accustomed to high-intensity exercise. But don't let this scare you off or stop you from continuing. Remind yourself that the soreness is only temporary, but the benefits of exercise, if you keep at it, are permanent.

BAD PAIN

Unlike DOMS, which tends to be dull and goes away after a few days, injury-related pain is typically sharp and may get worse with time. Also, it's usually confined to a specific location, which may hurt if you press the area or move it in a particular way.

Injuries can be acute, meaning they happen suddenly (a sprained ankle, for example), or they can be due to overuse (such as tennis elbow). Pulled muscles (also known as strains) and sprains, which are overextended or torn ligaments, are among the most common, but injuries can also come in other forms ranging from skin lesions to bone fractures. Though injuries can occur throughout the body, the areas most susceptible depend on your activity. For example, runners are especially prone to knee problems, shin splints, and plantar fasciitis (heel pain). Resistance training is more likely to lead to shoulder and back injuries.

At first glance, the prospect of all this misery may seem like a good reason to stay on the couch. Indeed, surveys show that the fear of injury is a common barrier to exercise, especially among older people. But that fear is misplaced. Exercise-related injury rates of older people are no higher than those of younger people, according to research. In addition, becoming stronger and more fit, at whatever age, may decrease your chances of getting injured from everyday activities and lead to less pain overall. (For more on how exercise can prevent back pain, see page 84.) These benefits, along with all the others described in chapter 2, easily outweigh the risk of injuries and pain from exercise.

While it's impossible to prevent injuries altogether, there are ways to reduce your chances of getting hurt. Here are 10 tips to keep in mind:

1. Warm up.

Doing light aerobic activity for a few minutes along with dynamic stretches gets your blood flowing and helps prepare muscles, tendons, ligaments, and joints for what's to come.

2. Use proper form.

If you're doing resistance or plyometric exercises in the *Fitter Faster* program, carefully follow the instructions in chapter 10. If you're not sure how to do an exercise, ask a fitness professional at a gym (if you belong to one) or look for a demonstration video online from a trusted source. Lifting weights in front of a mirror can help you make sure that all parts of your body are properly positioned and that you're performing the exercise correctly. Generally, you should keep your abs tight and your knees slightly bent while lifting. Avoid arching or straining your back. To avoid hurting your back when picking up weights, bend your knees, keep your back straight, and lift with your legs.

Proper walking technique (yes, there is such a thing) includes keeping your head up, back straight, shoulders relaxed, and abs tight. Bend your elbows and swing your arms. Walk "heel to toe," meaning you should land on your heel, roll forward onto the ball of your foot, and push off from your toes.

As for running, look ahead, not down. Stand up straight and lean slightly forward, but don't slouch. Keep your shoulders and hands relaxed, and swing your arms close to your body with your elbows bent at a 90-degree angle. Your stride should be relatively short, and your foot should land under your body, not in front of it.

3. Ease into a new routine.

While it's good to be gung-ho when you start a workout program, doing too much too soon can quickly sideline you with an injury. To avoid this, start out slowly, and gradually increase the intensity. For example, if you're not used to running, choose walking, not sprinting, as your HIIT activity. Similarly, if a weight is too heavy to lift for the recommended number of reps, drop down to a lighter one. Over time, you'll need to push yourself to get results, but as you're beginning it's wise to err on the side of caution.

4. Be aware of trouble spots.

If you have a problem area—say, a shoulder with a previous injury or a knee with arthritis—use extra caution when doing exercises that involve that particular joint or muscle group. Though it may be okay to exert yourself there (exercising arthritic joints can be beneficial, for example), check with a medical professional to find out which exercises are (and are not) safe for you to do so that you avoid reinjuring yourself or making a problem worse.

5. Listen to your body.

If you feel pain during exercise, don't push through it. Stop and take a break. The same goes if you feel dizzy, light-headed, or nauseated.

6. Use proper gear.

Wearing the right clothing and other gear can help prevent a number of potential problems. Though the list of what you need depends on your activity, here are some highlights: Choose comfortable shoes that are designed for your activity, and make sure they fit properly. Replace them regularly. Also, wear socks made of synthetic fibers, which are better than cotton for preventing blisters. To avoid a rash, wear clothing that wicks away sweat. If you swim, wear earplugs to avoid swimmer's ear. When lifting weights, you may want to use gloves to protect against calluses and blisters on your hands. To reduce your chances of a head injury, always wear a helmet when you go biking outside. If you exercise outdoors when it's dusk or dark, wear light-colored clothing and reflectors. (For more on gear, see chapter 4.)

7. Mix it up.

Doing the same exercises too frequently can increase your risk of overuse injuries. That's one reason why a balanced plan like the *Fitter Faster* program, which involves a different workout each day of the week, is a good idea. Building in rest days is also important to help give your body time to recover.

8. Avoid tobacco.

Everyone knows that smoking can cause a host of harmful effects that counteract the benefits of exercise. But what you may not know is that smokers are more prone to exercise-related injuries. One study, for example, found that Army recruits who smoked were 50 percent more likely to be injured during basic training than those who didn't smoke. And it's not just cigarettes that may have this effect. Other research in military recruits undergoing training has linked *smokeless* tobacco use to increased injury rates. Though the reasons aren't fully understood, the message is clear: Tobacco and exercise don't mix. If you use any form of tobacco, this is yet another reason why it's important to quit.

9. Get enough sleep.

Sleep deprivation increases the general risk of injuries, and research in teenage athletes has linked a chronic lack of sleep to greater odds of a sports injury. Besides impairing motor skills, being tired or sleepy can negatively affect thinking, awareness, and judgment, all of which can make you more prone to injure yourself. As a result, if you feel sleepy or extremely tired, it may be wise to avoid exercises such as weightlifting that require a higher level of concentration and instead do something simpler like walking. While taking the day off is also an option, don't let tiredness become a regular excuse to skip your workout. In fact, doing some type of exercise may perk you up.

10. Pay attention.

Injuries often happen simply because of carelessness. For example, the most common reason that weightlifters wind up in U.S. emergency rooms isn't overexertion, as you might expect; it's dropping weights on hands, feet, and other body parts. Treadmills are another leading cause of injury. It's not hard to lose your footing and fall off the machine if

Is running bad for your knees?

Over the years, plenty of people have warned me that my joints would someday pay the price for my years of jogging. I'm happy to report that the evidence does not back them up.

For example, a study that followed long-distance runners ages 50 and older for 18 years found that they were no more likely to develop osteoarthritis of the knee than non-runners. In another study, which surveyed former college swimmers and cross-country runners up to 55 years after graduation, the runners reported no more pain in their knees or hips than the swimmers did. Those who ran the most during or after college—measured in either miles or years—had no greater risk of osteoarthritis.

If anything, the research overall suggests that runners have a *lower* risk of joint problems. One possible reason is that running strengthens muscles, which means less pressure on joints. It may also prevent weight gain, which has the same effect.

Still, running isn't risk-free. It can raise the odds of arthritis for certain people, including those with a history of joint injuries. And it can lead to a host of short-term injuries ranging from blisters to shin splints. To reduce your risk of running-related problems, follow the previous 10 tips and try to run on surfaces that are even and have some give.

you're distracted by something—whether your cell phone, the display, the TV remote, or another person. Similarly, texting while you walk outdoors is an invitation to injury, as is listening to music that prevents you from hearing oncoming traffic. In short, whether you're exercising at home, in a gym, or outdoors, don't let your guard down; try to be mindful of what you're doing and what's around you at all times.

RICE TO THE RESCUE

If you wind up with an injury, you may be able to treat it with RICE—but not the kind you eat. RICE stands for rest, ice, compression, and elevation.

Rest: Stop using the affected area for a day or two and see if the injury gets better. Over time, however, too much rest can impede recovery, so you want to gradually start moving the area again as soon as the pain and swelling subside.

Ice: To reduce pain and swelling, apply ice to the area for about 20 minutes, several times a day. (Though evidence supporting the practice isn't ironclad, there's greater consensus about the benefits of ice for acute injuries than for DOMS.) You can use an ice pack, ice cubes in a sealable plastic bag, or even a frozen package of vegetables. Just be sure to place it in a damp towel so the ice doesn't hurt your skin.

Compression: Wrap the area in an elastic bandage to reduce swelling. Make it snug but not so tight that it causes numbness or tingling.

Elevation: Keep the area raised to a level at or above your heart. This may help decrease swelling by causing fluid to drain.

In addition, an NSAID can help reduce discomfort. As with all medications, however, take no more than the recommended amount, and use it for as short a time as possible.

If you're not improving after a few days, contact a health-care provider. Seek medical attention right away if you can't put any weight on the area or you think that a bone may be broken or a joint dislocated. The same goes if you have severe pain or bleeding.

As you're recovering, be patient and give yourself adequate time to heal before jumping completely back into your routine. If you try to do too much too quickly, you may reinjure yourself. At the same time, don't use an injury as an excuse to stop exercising. Instead, keep working areas of your body that aren't injured. If you have a shoulder injury, for example, do exercises involving your legs. If you have a foot injury, do resistance training for your upper body. And if you have to stop doing particular activities permanently, find others that you can do. Just don't let injuries put a permanent end to your exercise.

JUDY

AGE 51

FAIRFAX, VIRGINIA

Judy had every reason to believe she would accomplish big things as an athlete. An all-state female rugby player and Junior Olympian in rowing, Judy pushed herself and her body as hard as she could. Her regimen included a daily run followed by a jump-rope session that lasted at least 20 minutes. Seeing improvements in her endurance and strength, Judy continued to jump more and more, never missing a single day. "I even took my jump rope on road trips and requested ground-floor rooms so I could jump in hotels," she says.

The intense training paid off with a firm, trim body that could meet any physical challenge. Until it couldn't. Persistent pain that was unbearable sent her to doctors, and X-rays revealed bone-on-bone in both hips. All the activities she'd previously loved—especially jumping rope—were immediately off limits. "I was so excited about the immediate results I saw from jump-roping," Judy recalls, "it never occurred to me that the long-term damage would sideline me entirely."

Initially frustrated that she couldn't participate in her favorite activities and worried that she would fall out of shape, Judy researched low-impact exercises. A few weeks later, she grabbed some goggles and jumped into the pool. Swimming laps and doing water aerobics, Judy found a new way to maintain her previous level of challenging physical activity. It turns out that her injuries didn't require giving up exercise; she just had to make some adjustments. "Now, swimming helps me get out of bed in the morning," she says, "with no pain."

Get Going

The *Fitter Faster* Plan

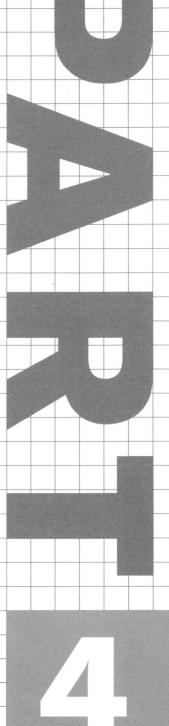

PART 4

The Workouts

Now it's time to put what you've learned into action. The *Fitter Faster* workout plan, designed in conjunction with personal trainer Brad Kolowich Jr. (who appears in the photos in this chapter, along with Mandy Malool), has six key features:

Time-Efficient: You'll be able to complete many of the workouts in as little as 15 minutes and get the same benefits that you would from more time-consuming regimens. Our routines are designed as accordions so that on days you have more time, you can lengthen your workouts and achieve even better results.

Comprehensive: Our program incorporates elements of a well-rounded exercise plan, including aerobic conditioning, strength training, plyometrics, and stretching, so you'll get everything you need here.

Varied: For five days a week, you'll have a different routine every day, which will keep you from getting bored. On the sixth day, you can choose whatever activity you wish. (Day 7 is for rest.)

Customizable: The plan includes routines for beginner, intermediate, and advanced exercisers, with progressively higher levels of difficulty and complexity. You can start at a level that's right for you and as your aerobic fitness and strength increase, move up and continue to challenge yourself. Also, for aerobic training (both conventional and HIIT), you can select which activities to do—based on what you enjoy or what's most convenient on a given day.

Convenient: The only equipment you'll need for the program is a set of dumbbells, which you can purchase online or at a sporting-goods store. On some days, you'll need no equipment. All the workouts can be done at home or outdoors. However, if you prefer exercising at a gym and using equipment there, you can certainly do so with this program.

Effective: Using these workouts, Brad has seen excellent results among clients of all shapes, sizes, ages, and fitness levels. With our plan you'll improve your endurance, increase your strength, tone your body, and perhaps shed fat. Most important, you'll get healthier overall.

KNOW THYSELF

Since our program involves high-intensity workout routines, it's important to get clearance first from a medical professional if you have a chronic condition such as heart disease, diabetes, or arthritis. The same goes if you've been sedentary or are new to exercise. The Physical Activity Readiness Questionnaire (PAR-Q), which you can find online, is a useful tool for determining whether you can safely begin an exercise program.

Once you're ready to start, you need to find out your baseline level of fitness, which is crucial for tracking your progress as you go forward. To that end, do these four tests, record the results, and then repeat the tests monthly. If you don't see the improvements that you want, try increasing the intensity of your workouts.

Push-Up

Lie face down with your body straight and your hands at about chest height and slightly outside of shoulder width. Straighten arms to lift yourself off the floor, keeping your back flat. Lower your body until your chest is two inches off the floor and then push back up to the arms-straight position. If you're unable to do a standard push-up, start with knees bent and touching the floor. Count how many you can do before failure.

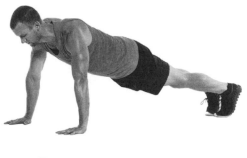

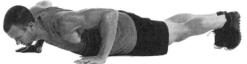

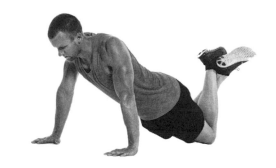

Half Sit-Up

Lie on your back with your knees bent and feet flat on the floor. Keep arms straight and on the floor beside your hips with your palms facing down. Flex at your waist to raise your upper torso off the floor as high as possible while keeping your lower back on the floor. Return to the starting position. Count how many you can do in 60 seconds.

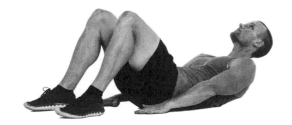

Bench Squat

Stand with feet shoulder width apart, arms crossed, and hands on shoulders with elbows in front of you. Squat down by bending at the hips and shifting your butt back while bending your knees. Continue movement downward until your upper legs are parallel to the floor and your butt touches a couch, chair, or bench. Keep your feet planted on the floor, your head and chest up, and your back straight. Stand up and return to the starting position. Count how many you can do in 60 seconds.

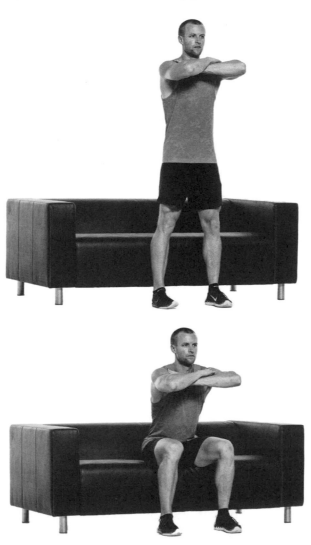

Heart Rate Recovery

Using the talk test described on page 66, walk or jog for 5 minutes at a pace at which you can speak without becoming breathless but can't sing. When you're done, measure your heart rate immediately by placing two fingertips (not a thumb) on the opposite wrist just below the base of your thumb. Count the number of beats for 10 seconds and multiply by 6. Wait two minutes and do the same thing again. Subtract the second reading from the first. As your aerobic fitness improves, your heart rate will return to normal more quickly, and the difference between the two numbers will increase.

Many people also find it useful to track body measurements, for which you'll need a tape measure. These include:

- Chest (circumference around the nipple line)
- Shoulders (around the widest part)
- Upper arms
- Waist (don't suck in your stomach!)
- Hips
- Upper legs
- Calves

One more thing you need to assess before starting is your experience level with exercise: beginner, intermediate, or advanced. If you're sedentary or haven't exercised in a while, go for the beginner regimens. If, on the other hand, you're accustomed to vigorous workouts and are in excellent shape, the advanced plans might be appropriate. Keep in mind that you may fall into different categories for aerobic and strength training. For example, if you walk or jog regularly but have little or no experience lifting weights, you might start with the intermediate program for aerobic exercise and the beginner program for strength training.

Because everyone is different and there's no one-size-fits-all test, you'll need to use your own judgment about where you fit. If you're uncertain, start at the beginner level. That way you can make sure that you're capable of doing the exercises and minimize the chances of injury. If you find that you're not challenged enough, you can always move up.

In general, we recommend sticking with a level for three months before moving to the next one (especially if you're a beginner). But everyone progresses differently, so it's fine if you move up more quickly or stay with the same level longer. If you do advance, make sure that you can do all the exercises at the next level properly and safely. If that's not the case, return to the previous level and stick with it until you're ready to try moving up again. And of course if you experience pain, nausea, lightheadedness, or dizziness at any level, stop immediately.

FITTER FASTER PROGRAM OVERVIEW

	WORKOUT	DESCRIPTION
Day 1	Strength Circuit 1	Eight exercises targeting chest, back, arms, shoulders, legs, and core. Exercises become more complex at higher levels. 15–20 minutes total*
Day 2	HIIT	Choose an activity such as walking, running, cycling, rowing, or stair climbing. High-intensity intervals last from 15 seconds to 1 minute depending on level. 15–20 minutes total
Day 3	Conventional Cardio	Choose any activity of moderate to vigorous intensity and do at a continuous rate for at least 10 minutes at a time. 35 minutes total
Day 4	Strength Circuit 2	Same as day 1 except with different exercises. 15–20 minutes total
Day 5	HIIT Plyometrics	Eight to 10 exercises (depending on level), each done for 30 seconds. Rest time between exercises declines as level increases. 15 minutes total
Day 6	Your Choice	Choose a routine from the plan, do a conventional cardio activity, or take a fitness class you enjoy.
Day 7**	Rest	After six days of workouts, you've earned it!

*Approximate total time includes one round of exercises along with warm-up and stretching or cool-down.

 **While we recommend performing the exercises in this order, it's fine to do them in a different order or to have your rest day occur at a different point in the week.

THE WORKOUTS

EXERCISE PLANS

WARM UP

As discussed in chapter 7, warming up will get your blood flowing and help you better perform the exercises. Begin every workout with the following routine, which should take less than five minutes.

1. Walk or jog

Walk or jog in place at a relatively low intensity (3 or 4 on a scale of 10) for two or three minutes.

2. Arm Circles

Stand and straighten arms out to your sides, making a giant "T." Form small circles forward for 15 reps. Repeat the same motion backward 15 times.

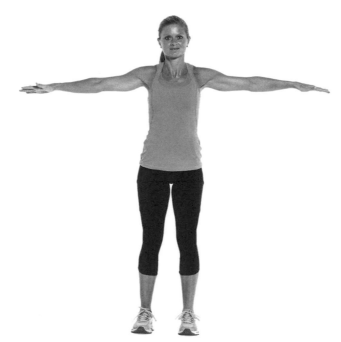

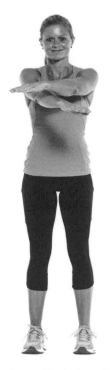
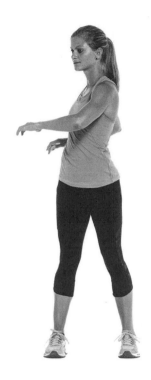

Cross-Body Arm Swing   Alternating Twist

3. Cross-Body Arm Swings

Stand and straighten arms out to your sides, forming a giant "T." Swing
arms across each other, alternating the arm that's on top. Do 16 swings.

4. Alternating Twist

Stand and twist your upper torso from side to side while letting your
arms swing freely. Twist to each side 15 times.

5. Leg Swings

Stand and support yourself with one arm against a wall or on a couch or chair. Swing leg on the other side forward and backward 15 times. Then brace yourself with the opposite arm and repeat with the other leg.

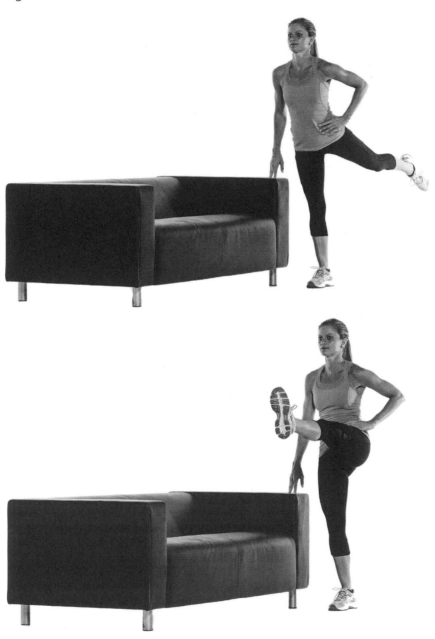

DAY 1: STRENGTH CIRCUIT 1

For this routine you'll need dumbbells, a couch or bench, and a step. Do each exercise in a controlled manner, focusing on proper form. And don't forget to breathe. Exhale as you lift the weight (or do the hardest work) and inhale as you lower it.

As you'll see, we change the rep counts monthly for the beginner level and weekly for intermediate and advanced levels. As discussed in chapter 6, varying the reps (an approach known as periodization) can help improve your results by keeping you from plateauing.

Choose a weight that gets you to failure within the rep range, meaning that you're unable do another rep after the last one. Once you can complete all reps with proper form, increase the weight by five pounds (or less if the dumbbells you're using come in smaller increments). Keep in mind that different exercises will require different weights. For exercises that don't involve weights, you'll sometimes be directed to do an exercise to failure.

Move as quickly as you can between exercises, resting for 30 seconds at most. A single round of the circuit is sufficient, but if you have additional time and want to push yourself more and achieve better results, complete two or three rounds. Stretch afterward with the exercises described on pages 162–165.

BEGINNER LEVEL

MONTH	1	2	3	4*	5	6
REPETITIONS	20	15	12	10	8	6

*Though we generally recommend sticking with a level for three months, rep counts for subsequent months are included in case you wish to continue longer at the beginner level.

1. Modified Push-Up

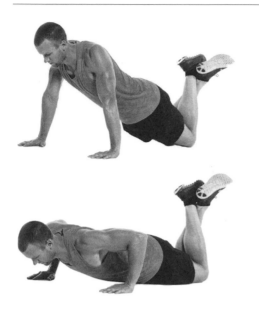

Lie face down with knees bent and palms on the floor at about chest height and just outside of shoulder width. Straighten arms to lift yourself off the floor, keeping your back flat. Lower your body until chest is as close to the floor as possible and then push back up. Do as many as you can until failure. For a bigger challenge, start with legs straight and feet on the floor.

2. Single-Arm Row

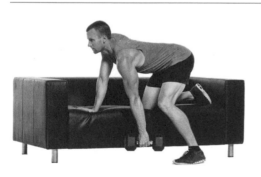

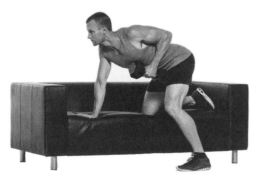

With your right side facing a couch or bench, place right knee and right hand on the seat. Leaving left foot planted and left knee slightly bent, grab dumbbell from the floor with palm facing the seat. Pull up until upper arm reaches parallel to floor or just slightly higher. Keep elbow close to your side and squeeze right shoulder blade toward your spine. Lower the dumbbell until arm is extended. Repeat with right arm. Do the recommended number of reps on each side.

3. Bodyweight Squat

Stand with feet shoulder width apart, arms crossed, and hands on shoulders with elbows in front of you. Bend at the hips and shift butt back while bending knees. Continue movement downward until upper legs are parallel to the floor. Keep feet planted on the floor, head and chest up, and back straight. Stand up and return to the starting position. Do as many squats as you can until failure. For a bigger challenge, hold a dumbbell tucked into the front of your chest throughout the movement.

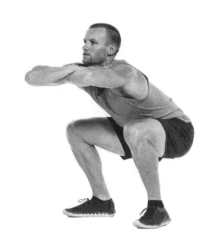

4. Overhead Shoulder Press

Standing with feet shoulder width apart and knees slightly bent, start with dumbbells raised to your ears, palms facing forward, and elbows at a 90-degree angle. Press upward until arms are fully extended above your head. Slowly lower to the start position.

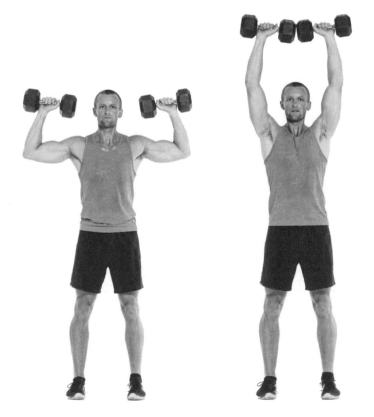

5. Hammer Curl

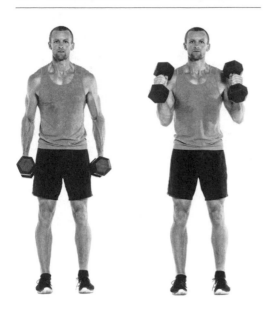

Stand holding dumbbells at your sides with palms facing each other. Keeping your elbows in, bend them to raise weights to your shoulders. Pause and then slowly lower the weights to the starting position.

6. Overhead Tricep Extension

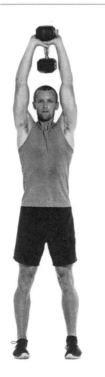
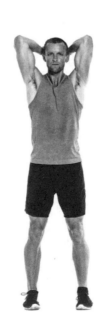

Stand upright with feet shoulder width apart and knees slightly bent. Holding a dumbbell with both hands, raise it over your head until arms are fully extended. Position palms so they face upward and the dumbbell hangs vertically from them. Lower the dumbbell behind your head until your elbows are fully bent. Keep elbows tucked in and pointed toward the ceiling. Press the dumbbell back up.

7. Calf Raise

Stand with legs straight. Grab a dumbbell in one hand and lift up onto the balls of both feet, raising heels as high as possible. Do half the recommended number of reps and then switch the dumbbell to the other hand and repeat.

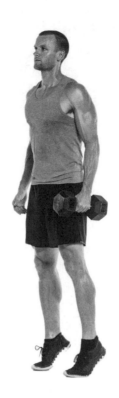

8. Crunch

Lie flat on your back with knees bent and feet flat on the floor. Cross hands over your chest. Flex at your waist to raise upper torso as high as possible while keeping low back on the floor. Return to the starting position, keeping your abdominal muscles under constant tension. Do as many reps as you can until failure.

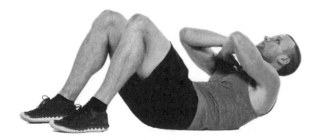

WEEK	1	2	3	4
REPETITIONS	18–20	14–16	10–12	6–8

After four weeks, repeat the cycle beginning at week 1 rep range.

1. Modified Decline Push-Up

Lie face down with your body straight and knees bent and elevated on a step, chair, couch, or bench. Place palms on the floor at about chest height and just outside of shoulder width. Straighten arms to lift yourself off the floor, keeping your back flat. Lower your body until chest is as close to the floor as possible and then push back up. Do as many as you can until failure. For a bigger challenge, start with legs straight and feet on the elevated surface.

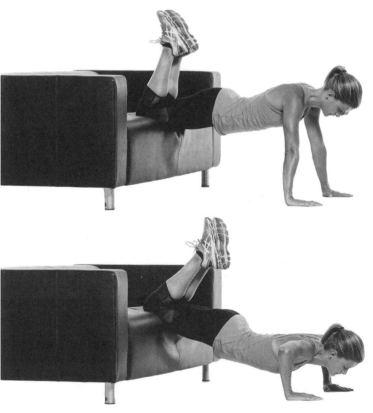

2. 45-Degree Bent-Over Row

Stand with feet shoulder width apart. Grab a dumbbell in each hand with knuckles facing forward. Bend knees slightly, keep your back straight, and lean forward at the hips at a 45-degree angle. Pull elbows back as you lift the dumbbells toward your belly button while squeezing shoulder blades together. Maintaining the 45-degree angle, lower the weights.

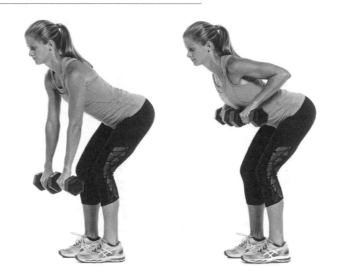

3. Walking Lunge

Stand while holding a dumbbell in each hand by your sides with palms facing each other. Take a large step forward and lower your body so back knee is bent and within an inch of the ground. Keep front knee behind your toes. Applying pressure on the ball of your back foot and the heel of your front foot, explode forward to the upright position. Repeat with leg positions reversed.

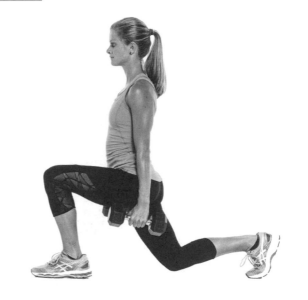

153

4. Squat to Overhead Press

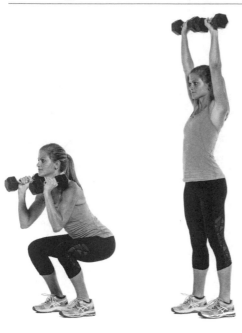

Stand upright with feet shoulder width apart and a dumbbell in each hand. Hold in front of your body at about head height with your elbows bent and palms facing each other. Bend at the knees and hips and squat down until your upper legs are parallel to the floor. Apply pressure through your heels and keep feet flat on the floor. Explode back up to the upright position while pressing the weights over your head until arms are fully extended. Rotate hands 90 degrees throughout the movement so that you finish with knuckles facing you. Return weights to head height.

5. Romanian Deadlift to Hammer Curl

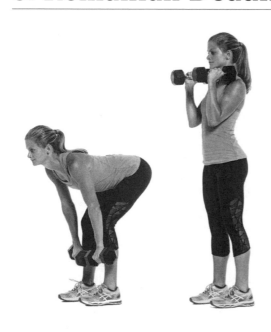

Stand with feet shoulder width apart. Hold a dumbbell in each hand with your knuckles facing forward. Initiate the deadlift by keeping your back straight and bending at the knees. Drive hips back as you lower the dumbbells toward the floor as far as possible, keeping dumbbells within an inch of your legs. Explode back up to the starting position, with the weights staying close to your legs and your back straight. Once in the upright position, rotate your hands so that your palms face each other. Keeping elbows in, bend them to raise the weights to your shoulders, contract your biceps, and then slowly lower the weights to the starting position.

6. Dual Overhead Tricep Extension

Stand with your feet shoulder width apart. Hold a dumbbell in each hand over your head, with palms facing each other and arms fully extended. Bending at the elbows, lower the dumbbells behind you while keeping elbows tucked in and pointing upward. Keeping the dumbbells separated, raise arms to starting position.

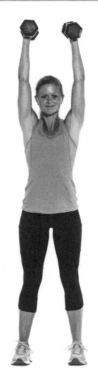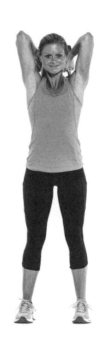

7. Alternating Elbow to Knee

Get in push-up position with your feet on the floor. Bring one knee to the opposite elbow, pause, and then return to the starting position. Repeat with the opposite leg. Do as many as you can until failure.

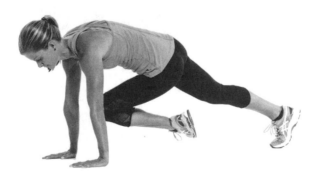

155

8. Calf Raise on Step

Stand with legs on a step so the balls of your feet are on the flat surface and heels are hanging over the edge. Grab a dumbbell in one hand and use the other hand to steady yourself. Drop heels until calves are fully stretched and then lift up onto the balls of feet, raising heels as high as possible. Do half the recommended number of reps and then switch the dumbbell to the other hand and repeat.

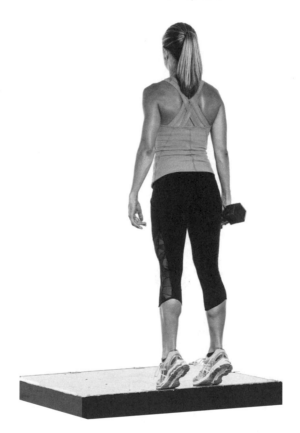

WEEK	1	2	3	4
REPETITIONS	16–18	12–14	8–10	4–6

After four weeks, repeat the cycle beginning at week 1 rep range.

1. Push-Up

Lie face down with your legs straight and feet on the floor. Place palms shoulder width apart at about chest height. Straighten arms to lift yourself off the floor, keeping your back flat. Lower your body until chest is as close to the floor as possible and then push back up. Do as many as you can until failure. For a bigger challenge, place hands close together.

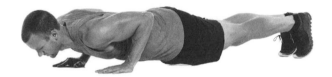

2. 90-Degree Bent-Over Row

Stand with feet shoulder width apart. Hold a dumbbell in each hand with knuckles facing forward. Bend knees slightly, keep your back straight, and lean forward at the hips at a 90-degree angle. Pull your elbows back as you lift the dumbbells toward your belly button while squeezing shoulder blades together. Maintaining the 90-degree angle, lower the weights.

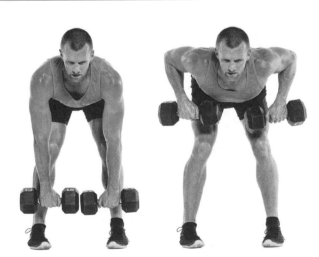

157

3. Romanian Deadlift

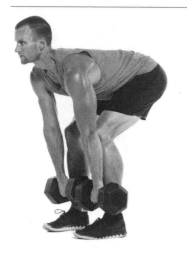

Stand with feet shoulder width apart. Hold a dumbbell in each hand with knuckles facing forward. Initiate the deadlift by keeping back straight and bending at the knees. Drive hips back as you lower the dumbbells toward the floor as far as possible, keeping dumbbells within an inch of your legs. Explode back up to the starting position with the weights staying close to your legs and your back straight.

4. Alternating Overhead Shoulder Press

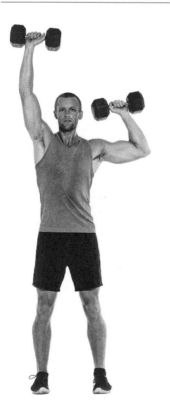

Standing with feet shoulder width apart and knees slightly bent, start with dumbbells raised to your ears, palms facing forward, and elbows at a 90-degree angle. Press one arm upward until it is fully extended above your head. Slowly lower to the start position. Then press the other arm up and lower. Repeat. Do the recommended number of reps on each side.

5. Walking Lunge to Zottman Curl

Stand while holding a dumbbell in each hand with palms facing each other. Take a large step forward and lower your body so that your back knee is bent and within an inch of the ground. Keep front knee behind your toes. Applying pressure on the ball of your back foot and the heel of your front foot, explode forward to the up-right position. Then, keeping your elbows in, initiate the bicep curl up by bending elbows to raise weights to your shoulders while rotating your wrists toward you. At the top of the curl, rotate wrists so palms face away from you. Pause and then slowly lower the weight with palms facing away. Repeat with leg positions reversed. Count each curl as one rep.

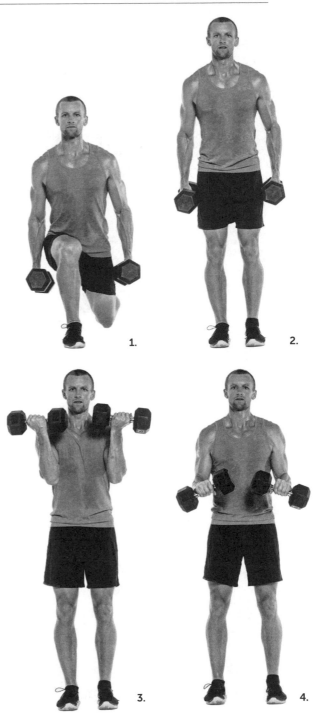

1.

2.

3.

4.

6. Squat to Overhead Press Extension

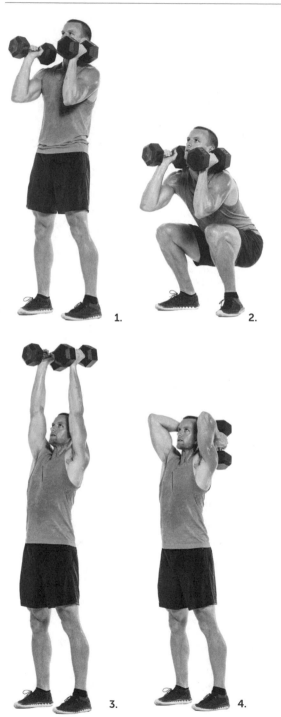

1.

2.

3.

4.

Stand with your feet shoulder width apart, holding a dumbbell in each hand at head height in front of you with elbows bent and palms facing each other. Bend at the hips and shift your butt back while bending your knees. Continue movement downward until upper legs are parallel to the floor. Keep feet planted on the floor, head and chest up, and back straight. Stand up while pressing dumbbells above your head until arms are straight with wrists continuing to face each other. At the top position, lower dumbbells behind your head until elbows are fully bent and then push back up until arms are fully extended again. Lower weights to the starting position.

7. Russian Twist

Sit on the floor and lean back at a 45-degree angle with knees bent and feet slightly elevated. Holding the weight with both hands in front of you, rotate upper torso from side to side. Count a rotation to both sides as one rep.

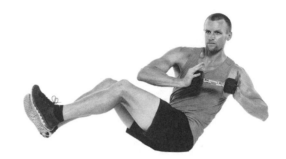

8. Single-Leg Calf Raise

Stand with legs straight on a step so that the balls of your feet are on the flat surface and heels are hanging over the edge. Grab a dumbbell in one hand and use the other hand to steady yourself. Bend knee of leg opposite to the dumbbell side so you're standing on one leg. Drop heel until calf is fully stretched and then raise up on your toes. Do the recommended number of reps and then repeat on the other leg, with the other hand holding the weight.

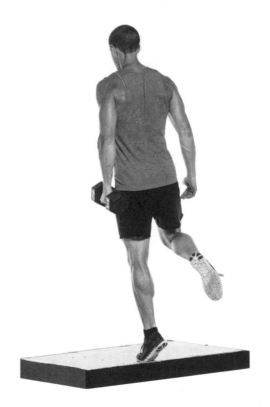

STRETCHING

After your routine, do the following stretches at least once (ideally twice or three times if you have extra time), holding each stretch for 20 to 30 seconds. Ease slowly into it and don't bounce. Remember to breathe.

1. Hamstring/Low-Back Stretch

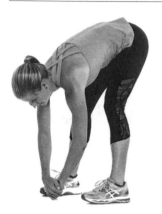

Stand with feet outside shoulder width and knees slightly bent. Lean forward at the hips until you feel a stretch in your lower back and the back of your legs.

2. Quad Stretch

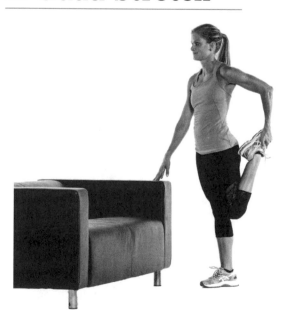

Hold on to a wall or piece of furniture with your right hand. Use left hand to grab right foot and pull up to your butt. Keep knees together. Hold, feeling stretch in your upper leg. Repeat with opposite hand and foot.

3. Glute/Back Stretch

Sit with your right leg straight and your left leg bent at the knee and across your right leg. Turn to your left and place your right elbow just outside your left knee, applying pressure to the outer knee. Hold and then do the same with the opposite side.

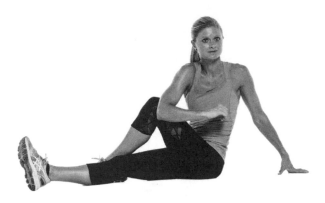

4. Chest Stretch

Stand with your feet shoulder width apart. Place hands behind neck with elbows flared out to your sides. Pull up and back with elbows to feel a stretch in your chest.

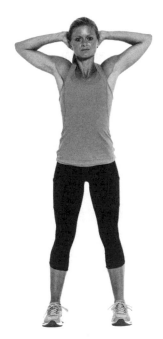

5. Tricep Stretch

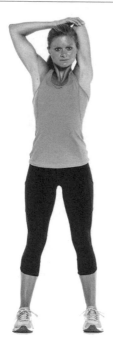

Stand with your feet shoulder width apart and left elbow bent and pointing up, staying close to your head. Grab elbow with right hand, push backward, and hold to feel a stretch in your upper arm. Repeat with opposite elbow and hand.

6. Shoulder Stretch

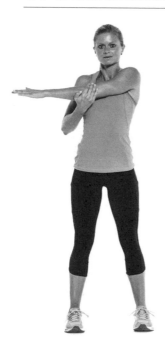

Stand with feet shoulder width apart and left arm straight across the front of your body. Pull on your left elbow with your right hand to feel a stretch in your shoulder. Hold and repeat with opposite arm and hand.

7. Calf Stretch

Place hands at about chest height on a wall. Facing wall, step back with one leg and forward with the other. Keep back leg straight, back foot flat and perpendicular to the wall, and front leg bent. Lean into the wall to feel a stretch in your back calf muscle. Hold and then do the same with your legs reversed.

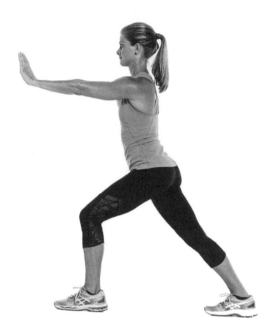

DAY 2: HIIT

Choose an activity such as walking, running, stair-climbing, rowing, cycling on a stationary bike, or using an elliptical machine that lends itself easily to interval training.

Do the warm-up routine on pages 144–146. Then alternate between intense intervals and moderately paced ones using the following guidelines.

BEGINNER LEVEL

Intense: 15 seconds at an intensity of 8 on a 10-point scale

Moderate: 45 seconds at an intensity of 5

Do 10 of each

INTERMEDIATE LEVEL

Intense: 30 seconds at an intensity of 9

Moderate: 30 seconds at an intensity of 5

Do 10 of each

ADVANCED LEVEL

Intense: 60 seconds at an intensity of 9

Moderate: 30 seconds at an intensity of 5

Do 10 of each

One round is fine, but if you have additional time and want even better results, do an additional round or two. When you're finished, cool down by doing your activity at a low intensity for 2 to 3 minutes. Add the stretching exercises on pages 162–165 if you have time.

DAY 3: CONVENTIONAL CARDIO

Choose an activity that you can sustain at an intensity that's moderate or vigorous (6 to 8 on a scale of 10) in increments of at least 10 minutes, for a total of 30 minutes. The activity can be an exercise such as walking, running, hiking, swimming, or biking. Or it can be a sport or pastime that you enjoy, like tennis, racquetball, basketball, volleyball, skiing, dancing, or playing with your kids. Household tasks like sweeping, vacuuming, mowing the lawn, raking leaves, and shoveling snow can count as well. (For more possibilities, see chapter 5.)

Begin with the warm-up on pages 144–146. When you're finished with the thirty minutes, cool down by walking or marching in place for two to three minutes. Add the stretching exercises on pages 162–165 if you have time.

DAY 4: STRENGTH CIRCUIT 2

Follow general instructions for Strength Circuit 1 (pages 147–161), including rep ranges for all levels, which are repeated below. Warm up (pages 148–150) beforehand and stretch (pages 166–165) afterward.

BEGINNER LEVEL

MONTH	1	2	3	4*	5	6
REPETITIONS	20	15	12	10	8	6

INTERMEDIATE LEVEL

WEEK	1	2	3	4
REPETITIONS	18–20	14–16	10–12	6–8

ADVANCED LEVEL

WEEK	1	2	3	4
REPETITIONS	16–18	12–14	8–10	4–6

1. Modified Incline Push-Up

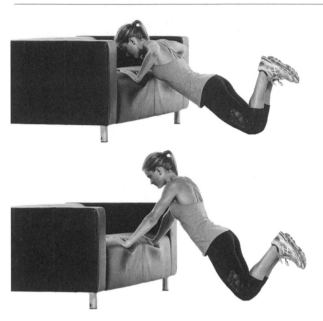

Lie face down in modified push-up position (see Day 1, Modified Push-Up.) Place your palms on an elevated surface such as a couch, chair, or stair step. Do as many push-ups as you can until failure. For a bigger challenge, start with legs straight and feet on the floor.

2. Floor Pullover

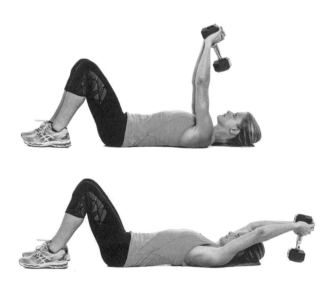

Lie on your back with knees bent and feet flat on the floor. Holding the dumbbell with both hands, raise it over your head with elbows slightly bent. Lower the weight in an arc behind your head until the dumbbell is about an inch from the floor. Raise the weight back to the starting position.

3. Alternating Reverse Lunge

Stand with your feet shoulder width apart, holding a dumbbell in each hand. Step backward with one leg while simultaneously bending your front leg until your front knee is at a 90-degree angle and parallel with your hip. Keep front knee behind your toes. Back knee should be just above the floor. Applying pressure on the ball of your back foot and the heel of your front foot, explode forward to the upright position. Repeat with the opposite leg. Do the recommended number of reps on each side.

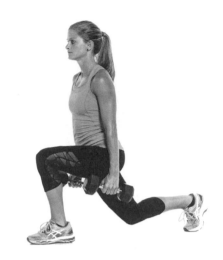

4. Upright Row

Stand with feet shoulder width apart. Grab a dumbbell in each hand with knuckles facing forward. Bend knees slightly, keep your back straight, and raise elbows to just above shoulder height while keeping the dumbbells close to your body. Slowly lower weights to the starting position.

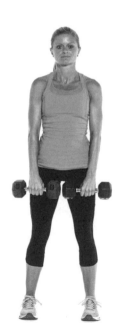
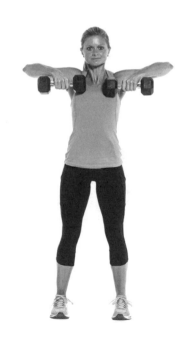

THE WORKOUTS

5. Bicep Curl

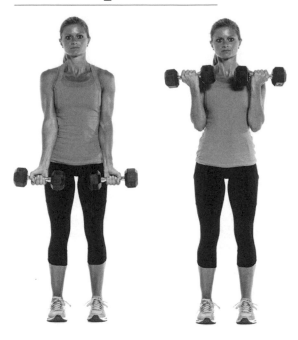

Stand holding dumbbells in front of your thighs with palms facing forward. Keeping your elbows in, bend them to raise weights to your shoulders. Pause and then slowly lower the weights to the starting position.

6. Floor Tricep Extension

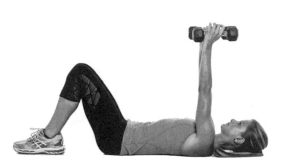

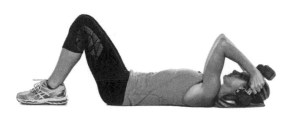

Lie on your back with knees bent and your feet flat on the floor. Hold a dumbbell in each hand over your head, with palms facing each other and arms fully extended. Bending at the elbows to just beyond 90 degrees, lower the dumbbells behind you while keeping your upper arms in a fixed position. Keeping the dumbbells separated, raise arms to starting position.

7. Reverse Crunch

Lie on your back with your knees bent and your feet flat on the floor. Move your knees up toward your chest and then raise your hips up off the floor, without relying on momentum to press up. Slowly return to the starting position. Do as many as you can until failure.

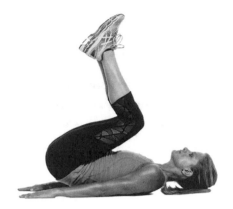

8. Superman

Lie face down on the floor with your arms and legs fully extended. Simultaneously raise your arms, legs, and chest up off the floor for a 1 to 2 second pause before slowly returning to the starting position. Do as many as you can until failure.

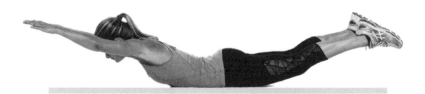

171

1. Push-Up

Lie face down with your legs straight and feet on the floor. Place palms on the floor at about chest height and just outside shoulder width. Straighten arms to lift yourself off the floor, keeping your back flat. Lower your body until chest is as close to the floor as possible and then push back up. Do as many as you can until failure.

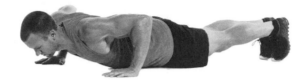

2. 45-Degree Bent-Over Row (reverse grip)

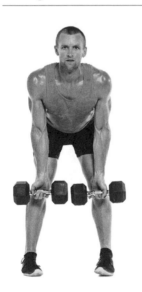
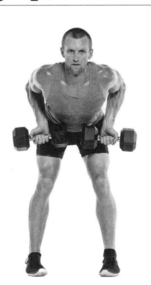

Stand with feet shoulder width apart. Grab a dumbbell in each hand with palms facing forward. Bend knees slightly, keep your back straight, and lean forward at the hips at a 45-degree angle. Pull elbows back as you lift the dumbbells toward your belly button while squeezing shoulder blades together. Maintaining the 45-degree angle, lower the weights.

3. Weighted Squat

Stand with your feet shoulder width apart and your arms at your sides with a dumbbell in each hand, palms facing each other. Bend at the hips and shift your butt back while bending knees. Continue movement downward until upper legs are parallel to the floor. Keep feet planted on the floor, head and chest up, and back straight. Stand up and return to the starting position.

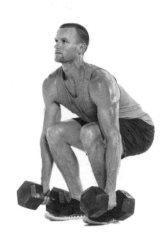

4. Romanian Deadlift to Upright Row

Stand with feet shoulder width apart. Hold a dumbbell in each hand with your knuckles facing forward. Initiate the deadlift by keeping your back straight and bending at the knees. Drive hips back as you lower the dumbbells toward the floor as far as possible, keeping dumbbells within an inch of your legs. Explode back up to the starting position with the weights staying close to your legs and your back straight. Once in the upright position, raise elbows to slightly above shoulder height while keeping the dumbbells close to your body. Slowly lower weights to the starting position.

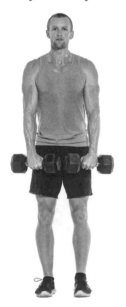
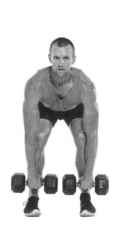
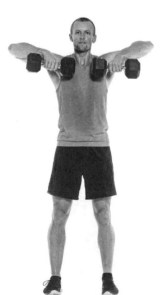

THE WORKOUTS

5. Rotating Wrist Bicep Curl

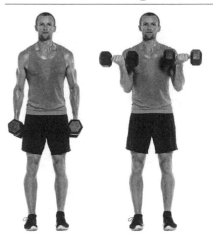

Stand holding dumbbells at your sides with palms facing each other. Keeping your elbows in, bend them to raise weights to your shoulders while rotating wrists so palms face up. Pause and then slowly lower the weights to the starting position.

6. Walking Lunge to Overhead Press Extension

Stand while holding a dumbbell in each hand at head height with palms facing each other. Keep elbows tucked in. Take a large step forward and lower your body so that your back knee is bent and within an inch of the ground. Keep front knee behind your toes. Applying pressure on the ball of your back foot and the heel of your front foot, explode forward to the upright position. Press the weights over your head until arms are fully extended with palms continuing to face each other. Then lower dumbbells behind your head until elbows are fully bent, and push back up again until arms are fully extended. Slowly lower weights to the starting position. This completes one rep. Repeat with leg positions reversed.

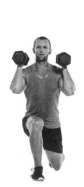
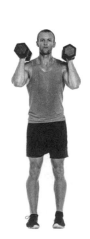
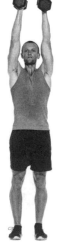
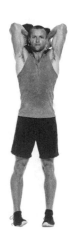

7. Bicycle

Lie on your back with your hands just behind your ears and your legs straight and slightly off the floor. Raise your right elbow and your left knee at the same time until they meet or come as close together as possible. Repeat with the opposite elbow and leg. Be careful not to pull your neck with your hands. Do as many reps as you can until failure.

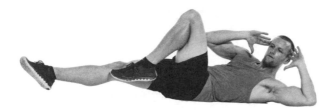

8. Birddog

Get on your hands and knees. Raise and extend left arm forward while simultaneously elevating and extending your right leg back and upwards. Hold for 1 or 2 seconds and then slowly return to the starting position. Repeat with the opposite arm and leg. Do the recommended number of reps on each side. For a bigger challenge, do the exercise on your hands and feet instead of your knees.

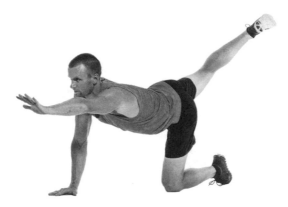

1. Reverse Grip Push-Up

Lie face down with legs straight and feet on the floor. Position dumbbells just below chest height at shoulder width. Place hands on weights with palms facing forward and get into arms-straight push-up position. Keeping elbows tucked in, lower your body until chest is as close to the floor as possible and then push back up. Do as many as you can until failure.

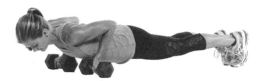

2. 90-Degree Bent-Over Row (neutral grip)

Stand with feet shoulder width apart. Hold a dumbbell in each hand by your sides with palms facing each other. Bend knees slightly, keep your back straight, and lean forward at the hips at a 90-degree angle. Pull your elbows back as you lift the dumbbells toward your belly button while squeezing shoulder blades together. Maintaining the 90-degree angle, lower the weights.

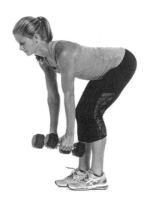
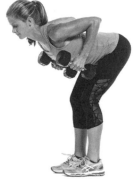

176

3. Single-Leg Squat

Stand on your left leg with right leg bent at the knee and behind you. Extend arms outward so they're parallel to the floor. Bend at the hips and shift your butt back while bending your left knee. Continue movement downward until upper left leg is parallel to the floor. Keep left foot planted on the floor, head and chest up, and back straight. Stand up by extending hips and left knee until you reach the upright position. Repeat with the other leg. Do the recommended number of reps on each side. For a bigger challenge, hold a dumbbell in front of your chest throughout the movement.

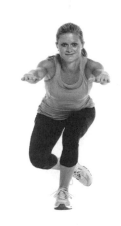

4. Walking Lunge to Arnold Shoulder Press

Stand while holding a dumbbell in each hand at about head height in front of you with palms facing you. Keep elbows tucked in. Take a large step forward and lower your body so that your back knee is bent and within an inch of the ground. Keep front knee behind your toes. Applying pressure on the ball of your back foot and the heel of your front foot, explode forward to the upright position. Then press the weights over your head until arms are fully extended. Rotate hands 180 degrees throughout the movement so that you finish with knuckles facing you. Return weights to the starting position at head height. Repeat with leg positions reversed. Count each shoulder press as one rep.

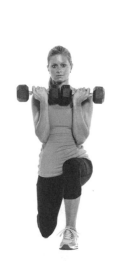
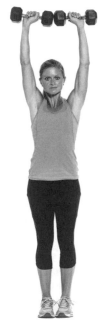

5. Squat to Hammer Curl

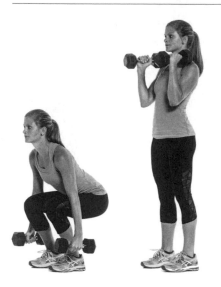

Stand with your feet shoulder width apart, holding a dumbbell in each hand by your sides with palms facing each other. Bend at the hips and shift your butt back while bending your knees. Continue movement downward until upper legs are parallel to the floor. Keep feet planted on the floor, head and chest up, and back straight. Stand up and then, keeping your elbows in, bend them to raise weights to your shoulders while keeping palms facing each other. Slowly lower the weights to the starting position.

6. Close-Grip Push-Up to Knee-In

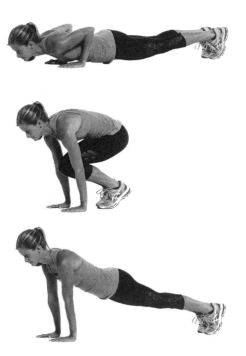

Get in push-up position with hands slightly closer than shoulder width apart. Keeping elbows tucked in, lower your body until chest is as close to the floor as possible, and push back up. Then, keeping feet together, drive knees to your chest, landing in a tucked position. Jump back to the starting position.

7. Romanian Deadlift to Bicep Curl to Shoulder Press

Stand with feet shoulder width apart. Hold a dumbbell in each hand with your palms facing forward. Initiate the deadlift by keeping your back straight and bending at the knees. Drive hips back as you lower the dumbbells toward the floor as far as possible, keeping dumbbells within an inch of your legs. Explode back up with the weights staying close to your legs and your back straight. Then curl the weight up to your shoulders with palms up and elbows locked into your side. Once at the top of the bicep curl, explode weights above your head, keeping palms facing you. Slowly lower weights to starting position.

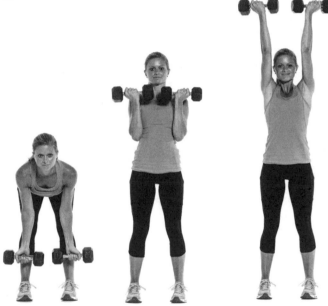

8. Good Morning

Begin by standing upright with knees slightly bent and a dumbbell resting on each shoulder. Keeping your back straight and shoulder blades together, bend at your hips and shift them back as you lean forward until your upper body reaches nearly parallel to the floor. Return to the starting position.

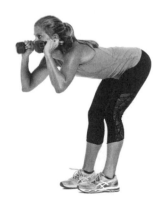

DAY 5: HIIT PLYOMETRICS

As discussed in chapter 6, plyometrics (jumping exercises) are effective for increasing power and strengthening bones. When done with high-intensity intervals, they're also an excellent aerobic workout.

All you need for this routine is a stopwatch or an app (such as one for Tabata) that allows you to set the work and rest times, along with the number of exercises. Do as many reps of each exercise as you can for 30 seconds, pushing yourself at an 8 or 9 on a scale of 10. Rest for the allotted time and then move to the next exercise. At higher levels, there are more exercises and shorter rest periods. One round is good; two or three are even better if you have the time.

As with the strength circuit, be sure to use proper form, and remember to breathe, exhaling as you do the hardest part of each exercise.

Warm up with the routine on pages 144–146, and do the stretching exercises on pages 162–165 afterward.

BEGINNER LEVEL
Rest for 30 seconds between each exercise.

1. Alternating Explosive Jump

Stand and explode one knee toward your chest as you jump up with the other leg. Land and repeat with legs switched.

2. Jumping Jack

Stand with your feet together and arms by your sides. Jump while simultaneously swinging arms upward over your head, with elbows slightly bent. Land with feet just outside of shoulder width. Jump back to starting position with arms by your sides.

3. Imaginary Jump Rope

Stand with feet together, knees slightly bent, and hands at your sides as if you are holding a jump rope. Mimic jumping rope by circling your wrists as you jump just a few inches off the floor.

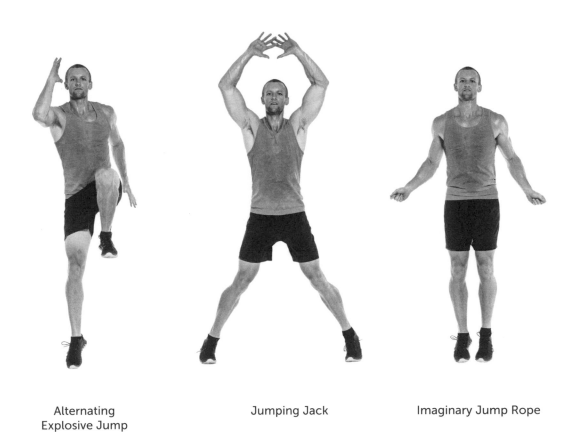

Alternating
Explosive Jump

Jumping Jack

Imaginary Jump Rope

4. Ski Jump

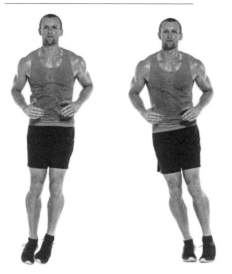

Stand with feet together and knees slightly bent. Jump explosively to one side with feet together. Once you land, quickly jump to the other side.

5. Scissor Jump

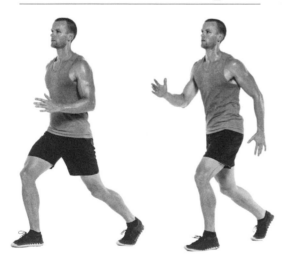

Stand with knees slightly bent with one leg forward and the other slightly behind you. Jump up and swing back leg forward and front leg backward. Repeat in an alternating movement.

6. Lateral Shuffle

Stand with your feet just outside shoulder width and knees bent. Then quickly shuffle two steps to your left followed by two steps back to your right. Repeat.

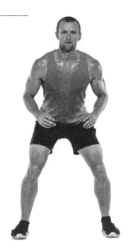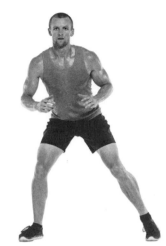

7. Run in Place

Stand with knees slightly bent and feet shoulder width apart. Drive one knee up followed by the opposite knee. Keep movements fast and explosive.

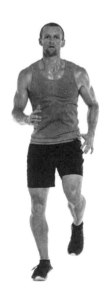

8. Alternating Punch

Stand with your knees slightly bent, elbows in, and hands by your face. Explosively extend one arm out in front of your body, quickly return it to the starting position, and repeat with the other arm.

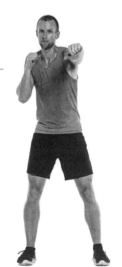

1. Power Jack

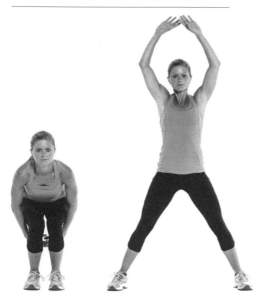

Stand with your feet together, hips back, knees bent, and back straight. Bend arms and place hands touching behind your legs. Jump and swing arms above your head, with a slight bend at the elbow. Land with feet just outside of shoulder width. Return to the starting position with arms underneath legs.

2. V Jump

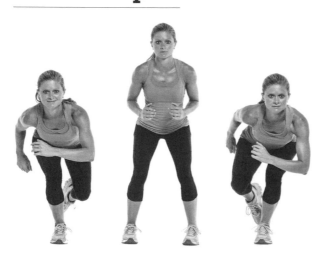

Stand with your feet shoulder width apart, knees slightly bent, and arms by your sides. Explosively jump diagonally forward to your right and land softly on your right foot. Immediately explode back to the starting position and then jump diagonally to your left and land on your left foot. Repeat, alternating sides.

3. Rocket Jump

Stand with your feet shoulder width apart. Squat down until upper legs are parallel to the floor or just slightly below. Explode up by thrusting arms toward the sky and jumping as high as you can. Land softly and drop back to the squat position.

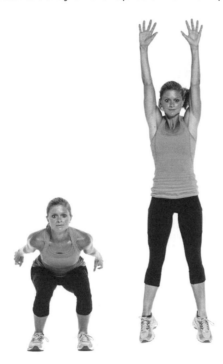

4. Butt Kick

Stand with feet shoulder width apart and knees slightly bent. Jump on one leg while simultaneously kicking the opposite heel back toward your butt. Land and repeat the same movement with the opposite leg.

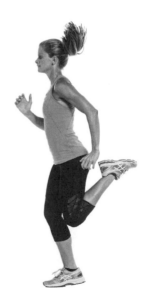

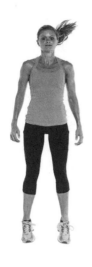

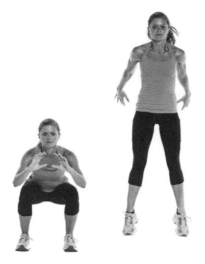

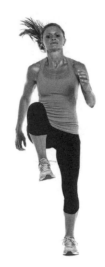

Calf Jump   Squat Jump   High Knee

5. Calf Jump

Stand with your feet shoulder width apart. Bend slightly at the knees and use calf muscles to explode up as high as you can. Land softly and repeat quickly.

6. Squat Jump

Stand with your feet shoulder width apart and arms in front of your body. Squat down until upper legs are parallel to the floor. Explode up off the ground and land softly with knees bent in a squat position.

7. High Knee

Stand with feet shoulder width apart and your knees slightly bent. Jump on one leg while simultaneously raising the opposite knee toward your chest. Land and repeat with the opposite leg.

8. Single Leg Hop

Stand on one leg with the other leg bent at the knee and foot behind you. Keeping your foot flat on the floor, bend at the knee and explode up. Land softly and repeat with the same leg for 15 seconds, switching to the other leg for the remaining 15 seconds.

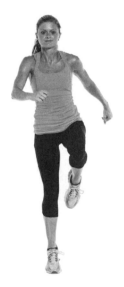

9. Mountain Climber

Start in push-up position with hands slightly outside of shoulder width. Explode one knee up to chest. Jump back to starting position while simultaneously exploding other knee to chest.

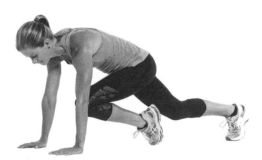

1. Burpee

Get in push-up position. Lower your body until your chest is as close to the floor as possible, and push back up. Then explode both knees up to your chest and drop into the bottom of a squat position, keeping feet flat on the floor and back straight. Jump up and land softly. Return to push-up position and repeat.

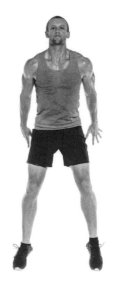

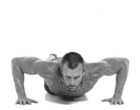
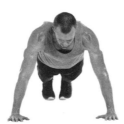
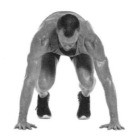

2. Speed Skater

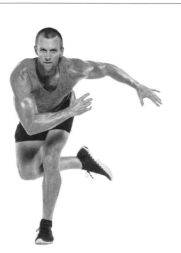

Balance on left leg in a crouched position with right foot up and behind you. Swinging arms in opposite directions to generate momentum, leap to the right and land on your right foot in a crouched position with left leg behind you. Land softly and repeat by leaping left.

3. Alternating-Stance Squat Jump

Stand with feet together and arms in front of your body. Squat down until upper legs are parallel to the floor. Explode up off the ground to the upright position, landing with feet outside of shoulder width. Repeat squat jump, but land with feet together. Alternate between two landing stances.

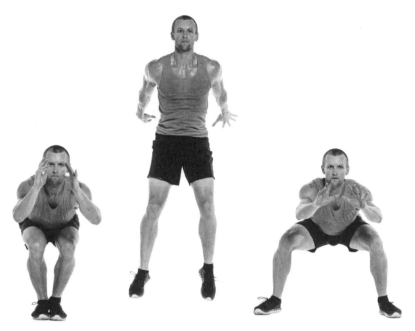

4. Switch Lunge

Begin at the bottom of the lunge position, with your front knee behind your toes and at a 90-degree angle. Jump straight up and switch legs while airborne. Land softly into the bottom of the lunge position with the opposite leg now forward. Repeat the movement in an alternating fashion.

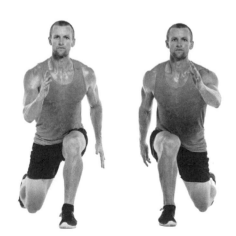

5. Tuck Jump

Stand with your feet shoulder width apart. Drop hips back slightly and bend at the knees while keeping feet flat on the floor. Explosively jump up as you tuck your knees up to your chest while airborne. Drop your knees back down, land softly, and then repeat.

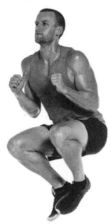

6. Push-Up Jack

Begin in push-up position. As you lower your body to the floor, explosively move your feet wider apart so they're outside of shoulder width. Push up explosively while jumping your feet to the starting position.

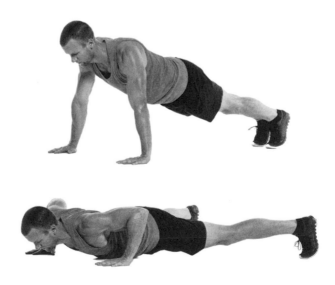

7. Hop Over

Keep your back straight and lean forward at the hips, forming close to a 90-degree angle. Hold on to a sturdy object such as a couch or bench. Explosively jump to the side with feet together as if you're jumping over a cone. Land softly with feet remaining together and then quickly jump in the opposite direction. Repeat.

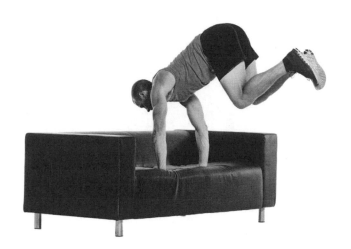

8. Explosive Long Jump

Stand with your feet just outside shoulder width, knees bent, and arms behind you. Swing your arms forward as you jump up and forward as far as possible. Land softly with your knees bent and immediately repeat.

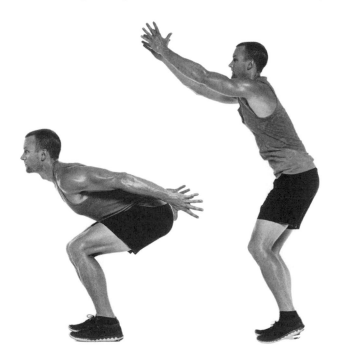

191

9. Alternating Plank Jump

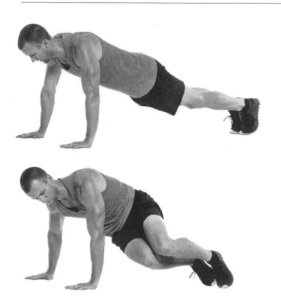

Get in push-up position. Explode both feet up together toward your left elbow. Jump feet back to the starting position and then explode both feet up toward your right elbow. Jump feet back to the starting position. Repeat.

10. 180-Degree Rotational Jumps

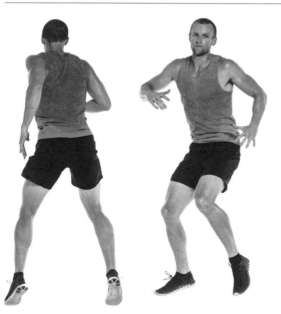

Stand with your knees bent and feet just outside of shoulder width. Drop hips slightly back, bend knees, and explosively jump up. Rotate your body 180 degrees while airborne so you land facing the opposite direction. Repeat going the opposite direction and land in the starting position.

DAY 6: YOUR CHOICE

Do HIIT, HIIT plyometrics, or one of the strength-training routines. Or select a conventional cardio activity and do it for a total of at least 30 minutes. Or take a fitness class you enjoy. Whatever you choose, be sure to warm up beforehand and cool down or stretch afterward.

PERSISTENCE PAYS

Once you're in an exercise routine, you'll inevitably have days when you feel as though your body is working in low gear and the exercises seem especially difficult. Don't let that discourage you; just do your best and expect that next time will be better.

Likewise, there may be days or weeks when you're unable to work out because of travel, illness, or family or work responsibilities. Don't let that become an excuse to quit. Even if you miss a few weeks, you won't lose all the improvements you've made. As soon as you're able, get moving again.

Fitness is a long-term endeavor and, as such, involves ups and downs. The key is to keep going despite the difficulties and distractions. I hope that what you've read in this book, including our time-saving workout plans, will make it easier to do so. Brad and I wish you all the best on what promises to be one of the most rewarding journeys of your life.

REFERENCES

CHAPTER 1

2 *survey by the Centers for Disease Control and Prevention:* Centers for Disease Control and Prevention. "Adult participation in aerobic and muscle-strengthening physical activities—United States, 011." *MMWR* 62.17 (2013): 326–330.

CHAPTER 2

9 *Jeremy Morris backed them up:* Morris, Jerry, et al. "Incidence and prediction of ischaemic heart-disease in London busmen." *Lancet* 288.7463 (1966): 553–559.

10 *elite athletes tend to live longer:* Garatachea, Nuria, et al. "Elite athletes live longer than the general population: A meta-analysis." *Mayo Clinic Proceedings* 89.9 (2014): 1195–1200.

10 *nine studies cumulatively involving more than 120,000 people:* Hupin, David, et al. "Even a low-dose of moderate-to-vigorous physical activity reduces mortality by 22% in adults aged ≥ 60 years: A systematic review and meta-analysis." *British Journal of Sports Medicine* 49.19 (2015): 1262–1267.

10 *study of more than 330,000 Europeans*: Ekelund, Ulf, et al. "Physical activity and all-cause mortality across levels of overall and abdominal adiposity in European men and women: The European Prospective Investigation into Cancer and Nutrition Study (EPIC)." *American Journal of Clinical Nutrition* 101.3 (2015): 613–621.

10 *Australian study:* Gebel, Klaus, et al. "Effect of moderate to vigorous physical activity on all-cause mortality in middle-aged and older Australians." *JAMA Internal Medicine* 175.6 (2015): 970–977.

10 *pooled results from 80 studies*: Samitz, Guenther, Matthias Egger, and Marcel Zwahlen. "Domains of physical activity and all-cause mortality: Systematic review and dose–response meta-analysis of cohort studies." *International Journal of Epidemiology* 40.5 (2011): 1382–1400.

11 *ooled results from six studies:* Moore, Steven, et al. "Leisure time physical activity of moderate to vigorous intensity and mortality: A large pooled cohort analysis." *PLoS Medicine* 9.11 (2012): e1001335.

11 *"compression of morbidity":* Willis, Benjamin, et al. "Midlife fitness and the development of chronic conditions in later life." *Archives of Internal Medicine* 172.17 (2012): 1333–1340.

12 *works its magic on the cardiovascular system:* Lin, Xiaochen, et al. "Effects of exercise training on cardiorespiratory fitness and biomarkers of cardiometabolic health: A systematic review and meta-analysis of randomized controlled trials." *Journal of the American Heart Association* 4.7 (2015): e002014; Lavie, Carl, et al. "Exercise and the cardiovascular system: Cinical science and cardiovascular outcomes." *Circulation Research* 117.2 (2015): 207–219.

12 *effect on the body's ability to use insulin:* Colberg, Sheri, et al. "Exercise and type 2 diabetes: The American College of Sports Medicine and the American Diabetes Association: joint position statement." *Diabetes Care* 33.12 (2010): e147–e167.

12 *exercisers who up their intensity:* Swain, David, and Barry Franklin. "Comparison of cardioprotective benefits of vigorous versus moderate intensity aerobic exercise." *American Journal of Cardiology* 97.1 (2006): 141–147.

12 *people with heart failure:* Ismail, Hashbullah, et al. "Clinical outcomes and cardiovascular responses to different exercise training intensities in patients with heart failure: A systematic review and meta-analysis." *JACC: Heart Failure* 1.6 (2013): 514–522.

12 *results from 52 studies:* Wolin, Kathleen Yaus, et al. "Physical activity and colon cancer prevention: A meta-analysis." *British Journal of Cancer* 100.4 (2009): 611–616.

13 *harmful effects of extreme exercise:* O'Keefe, James, et al. "Potential adverse cardiovascular effects from excessive endurance exercise." *Mayo Clinic Proceedings* 87.6 (2012): 587–595; Eijsvogels, Thijs, Antonio Fernandez, and Paul Thompson. "Are there deleterious cardiac effects of acute and chronic endurance exercise?" *Physiological Reviews* 96.1 (2016): 99–125.

13 *11 million participants:* Kim, Jonathan, et al. "Cardiac arrest during long-distance running races." *New England Journal of Medicine* 366.2 (2012): 130–140.

13 *American College of Sports Medicine:* Riebe, Deborah, et al. "Updating ACSM's recommendations for exercise preparticipation health screening." *Medicine & Science in Sports & Exercise* 47.11 (2015): 2473–2479.

14 *study of nearly 183,000 postmenopausal women:* Peters, Tricia, et al. "Physical activity and postmenopausal breast cancer risk in the NIH-AARP diet and health study." *Cancer Epidemiology Biomarkers & Prevention* 18.1 (2009): 289–296.

14 *other types of cancer:* Moore Steven, et al. "Association of leisure-time physical activity with risk of 26 types of cancer in 1.44 million adults." *JAMA Internal Medicine* 176.6 (2016): 816–825.

14 *well-established benefits:* Mutrie, Nanette, et al. "Five year follow up of participants in a randomized controlled trial showing benefits from exercise for breast cancer survivors during adjuvant treatment. Are there lasting effects?" *Journal of Cancer Survivorship* 6.4 (2012): 420–430; Mishra, Shiraz, et al. "Exercise interventions on

health-related quality of life for people with cancer during active treatment." *Cochrane Database of Systematic Reviews* 8 (2012): CD008465.

14 *may help extend the lives of cancer patients:* Je, Youjin, et al. "Association between physical activity and mortality in colorectal cancer: A meta-analysis of prospective cohort studies." *International Journal of Cancer* 133.8 (2013): 1905–1913; Ibrahim, Ezzeldin, and Abdelaziz Al-Homaidh. "Physical activity and survival after breast cancer diagnosis: Meta-analysis of published studies." *Medical Oncology* 28.3 (2011): 753–765.

14 *study that followed nearly 20,000 people:* DeFina, Laura, et al. "The association between midlife cardiorespiratory fitness levels and later-life dementia: A cohort study." *Annals of Internal Medicine* 158.3 (2013): 162–168.

14 *lower risk of dementia:* Beckett, Michael, Christopher Ardern, and Michael Rotondi. "A meta-analysis of prospective studies on the role of physical activity and the prevention of Alzheimer's disease in older adults." *BMC Geriatrics* 15 (2015): 9; Blondell, Sarah, Rachel Hammersley-Mather, and Lennert Veerman. "Does physical activity prevent cognitive decline and dementia? A systematic review and meta-analysis of longitudinal studies." *BMC Public Health* 14 (2014): 510.

14 *mild cognitive impairment*: Blondell, Sarah, Rachel Hammersley-Mather, and Lennert Veerman. "Does physical activity prevent cognitive decline and dementia? A systematic review and meta-analysis of longitudinal studies." *BMC Public Health* 14 (2014): 510.

15 *subjects randomly assigned to supervised exercise programs:* Groot, Colin, et al. "The effect of physical activity on cognitive function in patients with dementia: A meta-analysis of randomized control trials." *Ageing Research Reviews* 25 (2016): 13–23.

15 *single bout of exercise:* Weinberg, Lisa, et al. "A single bout of resistance exercise can enhance episodic memory performance." *Acta Psychologica* 153 (2014): 13–19.

15 *studies of middle-aged and older sedentary adults:* Smith, Patrick, et al. "Aerobic exercise and neurocognitive performance: A meta-analytic review of randomized controlled trials." *Psychosomatic Medicine* 72.3 (2010): 239–252.

15 *randomized trial of 120 older adults*: Erickson, Kirk, et al. "Exercise training increases size of hippocampus and improves memory." *Proceedings of the National Academy of Sciences* 108.7 (2011): 3017–3022.

15 *increase volume*: Colcombe, Stanley, et al. "Aerobic exercise training increases brain volume in aging humans." *Journal of Gerontology: Biological Sciences & Medical Sciences* 61.11 (2006): 1166–1170.

15 *levels of BDNF:* Ahlskog, Eric, et al. "Physical exercise as a preventive or disease-modifying treatment of dementia and brain aging." *Mayo Clinic Proceedings* 86.9 (2011): 876–884.

15 *needs to be moderately intense or vigorous:* Kirk-Sanchez, Neva, and Ellen McGough. "Physical exercise and cognitive performance in the elderly: Current perspectives." *Clinical Interventions in Aging* 9 (2014): 51–62.

15 *combination of aerobic exercise and strength training:* Smith, Patrick, et al. "Aerobic exercise and neurocognitive performance: A meta-analytic review of randomized controlled trials." *Psychosomatic Medicine* 72.3 (2010): 239–252.

16 *two dozen studies:* Mammen, George, and Guy Faulkner. "Physical activity and the prevention of depression." *American Journal of Preventive Medicine* 45.5 (2013): 649–657.

16 *followed 11,000 people over three decades:* Pereira, Snehal Pinto, Marie-Claude Geoffroy, and Christine Power. "Depressive symptoms and physical activity during 3 decades in adult life: Bidirectional associations in a prospective cohort study." *JAMA Psychiatry* 71.12 (2014): 1373–1380.

16 *review of 35 randomized trials:* Cooney, Gary, et al. "Exercise for depression." *Cochrane Database Systematic Reviews* 9 (2013): CD004366.

16 *alleviate anxiety:* Rebar, Amanda, et al. "A meta-meta-analysis of the effect of physical activity on depression and anxiety in non-clinical adult populations." *Health Psychology Review* 9.3 (2015): 366–378; Stonerock, Gregory, et al. "Exercise as treatment for anxiety: Systematic review and analysis." *Annals of Behavioral Medicine* 49.4 (2015): 542–556.

16 *enhanced sense of well-being:* Liao, Yue, Eleanor Shonkoff, and Genevieve Dunton. "The acute relationships between affect, physical feeling states, and physical activity in daily life: A review of current evidence." *Frontiers in Psychology* 6 (2015): 1975.

16 *"opens up the free flow of ideas":* Oppezzo, Marily, and Daniel Schwartz. "Give your ideas some legs: The positive effect of walking on creative thinking." *Journal of Experimental Psychology: Learning, Memory, and Cognition* 40.4 (2014): 1142–1152.

18 *review of 43 randomized studies:* Howe, Tracey, et al. "Exercise for preventing and treating osteoporosis in postmenopausal women." *Cochrane Database Systematic Reviews* 7 (2011): CD000333.

18 *studies show the same for men:* Bolam, Kate, Jannique Van Uffelen, and Dennis Taaffe. "The effect of physical exercise on bone density in middle-aged and older men: A systematic review." *Osteoporosis International* 24.11 (2013): 2749–2762.

18 *review of more than 120 randomized studies:* Liu, Chiung-ju, and Nancy Latham. "Progressive resistance strength training for improving physical function in older adults." *Cochrane Database Systematic Reviews* 3 (2009): CD002759.

18 *lower risk of falls:* Sherrington, Catherine, et al. "Effective exercise for the prevention of falls: A systematic review and meta-analysis." *Journal of the American Geriatrics Society* 56.12 (2008): 2234–2243.

18 *may reduce the risk of osteoarthritis:* Racunica, Tina, et al. "Effect of physical activity on articular knee joint structures in community-based adults." *Arthritis Care & Research* 57.7 (2007): 1261–1268.

18 *improve physical function and decrease joint pain:* Fransen, Marlene, et al. "Exer-

cise for osteoarthritis of the hip." *Cochrane Database Systematic Reviews* 4 (2014): CD007912; Fransen, Marlene, et al. "Exercise for osteoarthritis of the knee." *Cochrane Database Systematic Reviews* 1 (2015): CD004376.

18 *they don't have the deterioration:* Vopat, Bryan, et al. "The effects of fitness on the aging process." *Journal of the American Academy of Orthopaedic Surgeons* 22.9 (2014): 576–585.

18 *frail nursing home residents:* Fiatarone, Maria, et al. "Exercise training and nutritional supplementation for physical frailty in very elderly people." *New England Journal of Medicine* 330.25 (1994): 1769–1775.

19 *lower risk of erectile problems:* Hsiao, Wayland, et al. "Exercise is associated with better erectile function in men under 40 as evaluated by the International Index of Erectile Function." *Journal of Sexual Medicine* 9.2 (2012): 524–530; Simon, Ross, et al. "The association of exercise with both erectile and sexual function in black and white men." *Journal of Sexual Medicine* 12.5 (2015): 1202–1210.

19 *sedentary middle-aged men:* White, James, et al. "Enhanced sexual behavior in exercising men." *Archives of Sexual Behavior* 19.3 (1990): 193–209.

19 *research in women:* Cabral, Patrícia, et al. "Physical activity and sexual function in middle-aged women." *Revista da Associação Médica Brasileira* 60.1 (2014): 47–52.

19 *one unusual experiment:* Meston, Cindy, and Boris Gorzalka. "The effects of sympathetic activation on physiological and subjective sexual arousal in women." *Behaviour Research and Therapy* 33.6 (1995): 651–664.

20 *review of studies*: Stefani, Laura, et al. "Sexual activity before sports competition: A systematic review." *Frontiers in Physiology* 7 (2016): 246.

20 *involved former male athletes:* Johnson, Warren. "Muscular performance following coitus." *Journal of Sex Research* 4.3 (1968): 247–248.

20 *another study in male athletes*: Sztajzel, Juan, et al. "Effect of sexual activity on cycle ergometer stress test parameter, on plasmatic testosterone levels and on concentration capacity." *Journal of Sports Medicine and Physical Fitness* 40.3 (2000): 233–239.

21 *survey by the National Sleep Foundation: Sleep in America* poll, National Sleep Foundation (2013).

21 *review of 66 studies:* Kredlow, Alexandra, et al. "The effects of physical activity on sleep: A meta-analytic review." *Journal of Behavioral Medicine* 38.3 (2015): 427–449.

21 *small study of young adults*: Myllymäki, Tero, et al. "Effects of vigorous late-night exercise on sleep quality and cardiac autonomic activity." *Journal of Sleep Research* 20.1 pt. 2 (2011): 146–153.

21 *study in elderly people:* Benloucif, Susan, et al. "Morning or evening activity improves neuropsychological performance and subjective sleep quality in older adults." *Sleep* 27.8 (2004): 1542–1551.

21 *study that followed 1,000 adults:* Nieman, David, et al. "Upper respiratory tract

infection is reduced in physically fit and active adults." *British Journal of Sports Medicine* 45.12 (2011): 987–992.

22 *randomized trials on exercise and colds:* Lee, Hyun Kun, et al. "The effect of exercise on prevention of the common cold: A meta-analysis of randomized controlled trial studies." *Korean Journal of Family Medicine* 35.3 (2014): 119–126.

22 *experiment involving sedentary postmenopausal women:* Chubak, Jessica, et al. "Moderate-intensity exercise reduces the incidence of colds among postmenopausal women." *American Journal of Medicine* 119.11 (2006): 937–942.

22 *runners who participated in a Los Angeles marathon:* Nieman, David, et al. "Infectious episodes in runners before and after the Los Angeles Marathon." *Journal of Sports Medicine and Physical Fitness* 30.3 (1990): 316–328.

22 *review of more than 20 studies:* Steffens, Daniel, et al. "Prevention of low back pain: A systematic review and meta-analysis." *JAMA Internal Medicine* 176.2 (2016): 199–208.

23 *spraying a cold virus into their noses:* Weidner, Thomas, et al. "The effect of exercise training on the severity and duration of a viral upper respiratory illness." *Medicine and Science in Sports and Exercise* 30.11 (1998): 1578–1583.

24 *study of nearly 50,000 runners:* Williams, Paul. "Walking and running are associated with similar reductions in cataract risk." *Medicine and Science in Sports and Exercise* 45.6 (2013): 1089–1096.

24 *similar benefit regarding age-related macular degeneration:* Williams, Paul. "Prospective study of incident age-related macular degeneration in relation to vigorous physical activity during a 7-year follow-up." *Investigative Ophthalmology & Visual Science* 50.1 (2009): 101–106.

24 *followed roughly 4,000 people for 15 years:* Knudtson, Michael, Ronald Klein, and Barbara Klein. "Physical activity and the 15-year cumulative incidence of age-related macular degeneration: The Beaver Dam Eye Study." *British Journal of Ophthalmology* 90.12 (2006): 1461–1463.

24 *linked to risk factors for cardiovascular disease*: Du, Ya-Ru, et al. "Influence of metabolic syndrome on cataract risk: A meta-analysis of observational studies." *International Journal of Clinical and Experimental Medicine* 9.2 (2016): 1931–1941; Maralani, Haleh Ghaem, et al. "Metabolic syndrome and risk of age-related macular degeneration." *Retina* 35.3 (2015): 459–466.

24 *people who are overweight or obese are more prone*: Ye, Juan, et al. "Body mass index and risk of age-related cataract: A meta-analysis of prospective cohort studies." *PloS One* 9.2 (2014): e89923; Zhang, Qian-Yu, et al. "Overweight, obesity, and risk of age-related macular degeneration." *Investigative Ophthalmology & Visual Science* 57.3 (2016): 1276–1283.

25 *study of more than 68,000 female nurses:* Curhan, Sharon, et al. "Body mass index, waist circumference, physical activity, and risk of hearing loss in women." *American Journal of Medicine* 126.12 (2013): 1142.e1–8.

25 *linked higher fitness levels with better hearing:* Hutchinson, Kathleen, Helaine Alessio, and Rachael Baiduc. "Association between cardiovascular health and hearing function: Pure-tone and distortion product otoacoustic emission measures." *American Journal of Audiology* 19.1 (2010): 26–35; Loprinzi, Paul, Bradley Cardinal, and Ben Gilham. "Association between cardiorespiratory fitness and hearing sensitivity." *American Journal of Audiology* 21.1 (2012): 33–40.

25 *people cranked up the volume:* Hodgetts, William, Ryan Szarko, and Jana Rieger. "What is the influence of background noise and exercise on the listening levels of iPod users?" *International Journal of Audiology* 48.12 (2009): 825–832.

25 *study of middle-aged female nurses:* Townsend, Mary, et al. "Physical activity and incident urinary incontinence in middle-aged women." *Journal of Urology* 179.3 (2008): 1012–1017.

26 *study of older nurses:* Danforth, Kim, et al. "Physical activity and urinary incontinence among healthy, older women." *Obstetrics & Gynecology* 109.3 (2007): 721–727.

26 *study of men with BPH:* Wolin, Kathleen, et al. "Physical activity and benign prostatic hyperplasia–related outcomes and nocturia." *Medicine & Science in Sports & Exercise* 47.3 (2015): 581–592.

26 *study of sedentary older men:* Sugaya, Kimio, et al. "Effects of walking exercise on nocturia in the elderly." *Biomedical Research* 28.2 (2007): 101–105.

26 *study of 62,000 women:* Dukas, Laurent, Walter Willett, and Edward Giovannucci. "Association between physical activity, fiber intake, and other lifestyle variables and constipation in a study of women." *American Journal of Gastroenterology* 98.8 (2003): 1790–1796.

26 *trial involving inactive, middle-aged men and women:* De Schryver, Anneke, et al. "Effects of regular physical activity on defecation pattern in middle-aged patients complaining of chronic constipation." *Scandinavian Journal of Gastroenterology* 40.4 (2005): 422–429.

26 *study that followed participants for 20 years:* Hankinson, Arlene, et al. "Maintaining a high physical activity level over 20 years and weight gain." *JAMA* 304.23 (2010): 2603–2610.

27 *National Weight Control Registry:* Catenacci, Victoria, et al. "Physical activity patterns in the National Weight Control Registry." *Obesity* 16.1 (2008): 153–161.

27 *maintaining weight loss after 24 months:* Jakicic, John, et al. "Effect of exercise on 24-month weight loss maintenance in overweight women." *Archives of Internal Medicine* 168.14 (2008): 1550–1559.

27 *typically has little effect*: Swift, Damon, et al. "The role of exercise and physical activity in weight loss and maintenance." *Progress in Cardiovascular Diseases* 56.4 (2014): 441–447; Johns, David, et al. "Diet or exercise interventions vs. combined behavioral weight management programs: A systematic review and meta-analysis of direct comparisons." *Journal of the Academy of Nutrition and Dietetics* 114.10 (2014): 1557–1568.

28 *pooling results from more than 40 studies:* Biswas, Aviroop, et al. "Sedentary time and its association with risk for disease incidence, mortality, and hospitalization in adults: A systematic review and meta-analysis." *Annals of Internal Medicine* 162.2 (2015): 123–132.

29 *may make us hungrier:* King, Neil, et al. "Dual-process action of exercise on appetite control: Increase in orexigenic drive but improvement in meal-induced satiety." *American Journal of Clinical Nutrition* 90.4 (2009): 921–927.

29 *people who are overweight and fit live longer:* Fogelholm, Mikael. "Physical activity, fitness and fatness:Relations to mortality, morbidity and disease risk factors. A systematic review." *Obesity Reviews* 11.3 (2010): 202–221.

CHAPTER 3

32 *study of middle-aged women:* Segar, Michelle, Jacquelynne Eccles, and Caroline Richardson. "Rebranding exercise: Closing the gap between values and behavior." *International Journal of Behavioral Nutrition and Physical Activity* 8.94 (2011): 21884579.

34 *greater enjoyment from outdoor activities*: Coon, Thompson, et al. "Does participating in physical activity in outdoor natural environments have a greater effect on physical and mental wellbeing than physical activity indoors? A systematic review." *Environmental Science & Technology* 45.5 (2011): 1761–1772.

35 *we perform best at exercise:* Hill, David. "Morning-evening differences in response to exhaustive severe-intensity exercise." *Applied Physiology, Nutrition and Metabolism* 39.2 (2014): 248–254.

35 *athletes who train in the morning:* Chtourou, Hamdi, and Nizar Souissi. "The effect of training at a specific time of day: A review." *Journal of Strength and Conditioning Research* 26.7 (2012): 1984–2005.

36 *"forecasting myopia"*: Ruby, Matthew, et al. "The invisible benefits of exercise." *Health Psychology* 30.1 (2011): 67–74.

36 *randomized study of two such apps:* Cowdery, Joan, et al. "Exergame apps and physical activity: The results of the ZOMBIE trial." *American Journal of Health Education* 46.4 (2015): 216–222.

36 *large body of research*: Karageorghis, Costas, and David-Lee Priest. "Music in the exercise domain: A review and synthesis (part I)." *International Review of Sport and Exercise Psychology* 5.1 (2012): 44–66; Karageorghis, Costas, and David-Lee Priest. "Music in the exercise domain: A review and synthesis (part II)." *International Review of Sport and Exercise Psychology* 5.1 (2012): 67–84.

38 *"type of legal performance-enhancing drug":* Jabr, Ferris. "Let's get physical: The psychology of effective workout music." *Scientific American* March 30 (2013).

38 *tunes with 125 to 140 beats per minute:* Karageorghis, Costas, et al. "Revisiting the relationship between exercise heart rate and music tempo preference." *Research Quarterly for Exercise and Sport* 82.2 (2011): 274–284.

38 *people who participate in walking groups:* Kassavou, Aikaterini, Andrew Turner, and David French. "Do interventions to promote walking in groups increase physical activity? A meta-analysis." *International Journal of Behavioral Nutrition and Physical Activity* 10 (2013): 18.

39 *one involving 58 college-age women:* Irwin, Brandon, et al. "Aerobic exercise is promoted when individual performance affects the group: A test of the Kohler motivation gain effect." *Annals of Behavioral Medicine* 44.2 (2012): 151–159.

39 *web-based walking program:* Richardson, Caroline, et al. "An online community improves adherence in an internet-mediated walking program. Part 1: Results of a randomized controlled trial." *Journal of Medical Internet Research* 12.4 (2010): e71.

40 *more likely to become obese:* Christakis, Nicholas, and James Fowler. "The spread of obesity in a large social network over 32 years." *New England Journal of Medicine* 357.4 (2007): 370–379.

40 *smoker's chances of quitting:* Christakis, Nicholas, and James Fowler. "The collective dynamics of smoking in a large social network." *New England Journal of Medicine* 358.21 (2008): 2249–2258.

40 *study of 3,800 residents of New York City:* Firestone, Melanie, et al. "Perceptions and the role of group exercise among New York City adults, 2010–2011: An examination of interpersonal factors and leisure-time physical activity." *Preventive Medicine* 72 (2015): 50–55.

41 *3,300 heterosexual married couples:* Cobb, Laura, et al. "Spousal influence on physical activity in middle-aged and older adults: The ARIC study." *American Journal of Epidemiology* 183.5 (2016): 444–451.

41 *review of 11 randomized studies:* Mitchell, Marc, et al. "Financial incentives for exercise adherence in adults: Systematic review and meta-analysis." *American Journal of Preventive Medicine* 45.5 (2013): 658–667.

41 *goal of reaching 7,000 steps:* Patel, Mitesh, et al. "Framing financial incentives to increase physical activity among overweight and obese adults." *Annals of Internal Medicine* 164.6 (2016): 385–394.

42 *employees of a large company:* Royer, Heather, Mark Stehr, and Justin Sydnor. "Incentives, commitments and habit formation in exercise: Evidence from a field experiment with workers at a Fortune-500 company." 18580. National Bureau of Economic Research (2012).

43 *rats in cages with running wheels:* Roberts, Michael, et al. "Phenotypic and molecular differences between rats selectively bred to voluntarily run high vs. low nightly distances." *American Journal of Physiology—Regulatory, Integrative and Comparative Physiology* 304.11 (2013): R1024–R1035.

44 *data from 37,000 twin pairs:* Stubbe, Janine, et al. "Genetic influences on exercise participation in 37.051 twin pairs from seven countries." *PloS One* 1.1 (2006): e22.

44 *No Sweat:* Segar, Michelle. *No Sweat: How the Simple Science of Motivation Can Bring You a Lifetime of Fitness.* AMACOM (2015).

CHAPTER 4

46 *study of more than 900 novice runners:* Nielsen, Rasmus Oestergaard, et al. "Foot pronation is not associated with increased injury risk in novice runners wearing a neutral shoe: A 1-year prospective cohort study." *British Journal of Sports Medicine* 48.6 (2014): 440–447.

46 *research among military recruits:* Knapik, Joseph, et al. "Effect on injuries of assigning shoes based on foot shape in Air Force basic training." *American Journal of Preventive Medicine* 38.1 (2010): S197–S211; Knapik, Joseph, et al. "Injury reduction effectiveness of assigning running shoes based on plantar shape in Marine Corps basic training." *American Journal of Sports Medicine* 38.9 (2010): 1759–1767; Knapik, Joseph, et al. "Injury reduction effectiveness of selecting running shoes based on plantar shape." *Journal of Strength and Conditioning Research* 23.3 (2009): 685–697.

46 *researchers who reviewed the evidence:* Nigg, Benno, et al. "Running shoes and running injuries: Mythbusting and a proposal for two new paradigms: 'Preferred movement path' and 'comfort filter.'" *British Journal of Sports Medicine* 49.20 (2015): 1290–1294.

46 *biomechanics of running change:* Perkins, Kyle, William Hanney, and Carey Rothschild. "The risks and benefits of running barefoot or in minimalist shoes: A systematic review." *Sports Health: A Multidisciplinary Approach* 6.6 (2014): 475–480.

47 *may increase the risk of others:* Ridge, Sarah, et al. "Foot bone marrow edema after 10-week transition to minimalist running shoes." *Medicine & Science in Sports & Exercise* 45.7 (2013): 1363–1368.

47 *study by the American Council on Exercise:* Porcari, John, et al. "Will toning shoes really give you a better body?" American Council on Exercise (2010).

47 *shoes may increase the risk of injuries:* Maffiuletti, Nicola. "Increased lower limb muscle activity induced by wearing MBT shoes: Physiological benefits and potential concerns." *Footwear Science* 4.2 (2012): 123–129.

48 *researchers collected the sweaty shirts:* Callewaert, Chris, et al. "Microbial odor profile of polyester and cotton clothes after a fitness session." *Applied and Environmental Microbiology* 80.21 (2014): 6611–6619.

48 *clothing may not work as well as promised:* Walter, Nancy, Rachel McQueen, and Monika Keelan. "In vivo assessment of antimicrobial-treated textiles on skin microflora." *International Journal of Clothing Science and Technology* 26.4 (2014): 330–342.

48 *may come out in the wash:* Geranio, Luca, Manfred Heuberger, and Bernd Nowack. "The behavior of silver nanotextiles during washing." *Environmental Science & Technology* 43.21 (2009): 8113–8118.

50 *may pose a health risk:* Von Goetz, Natalie, et al. "Migration of Ag-and TiO2-(Nano) particles from textiles into artificial sweat under physical stress: Experiments and exposure modeling." *Environmental Science & Technology* 47.17 (2013): 9979–9987.

50 *garments may have small effects:* Born, Dennis-Peter, Billy Sperlich, and Hans-Christer Holmberg. "Bringing light into the dark: Effects of compression clothing on performance and recovery." *International Journal of Sports Physiology and Performance* 8.1 (2013): 4–18.

50 *review of 32 studies:* Engel, Florian Azad, Hans-Christer Holmberg, and Billy Sperlich. "Is there evidence that runners can benefit from wearing compression clothing?" *Sports Medicine* (2016): 1–14.

50 *reduce post-exercise muscle soreness and swelling:* Marqués-Jiménez, Diego, et al. "Are compression garments effective for the recovery of exercise-induced muscle damage? A systematic review with meta-analysis." *Physiology & Behavior* 153 (2016): 133–148.

51 *"the longer an athlete can wear compression":* Marqués-Jiménez, Diego, et al. "Are compression garments effective for the recovery of exercise-induced muscle damage? A systematic review with meta-analysis." *Physiology & Behavior* 153 (2016): 147.

53 *pole-walking benefits:* Pérez-Soriano, Pedro, et al. "Nordic walking: A systematic review." *European Journal of Human Movement* 33 (2014): 26–45.

56 *increasing the incline slightly:* Jones, Andrew, and Jonathan Doust. "A 1% treadmill grade most accurately reflects the energetic cost of outdoor running." *Journal of Sports Sciences* 14.4 (1996): 321–327.

57 *Consumer Reports recommends warranties*: "Treadmill buying guide: Fast track to buying a treadmill." (2016); "Elliptical buying guide: Tracking down the perfect machine." (2016); "Exercise bike buying guide: Pedal power." *Consumer Reports*, (2016).

57 *increases levels of physical activity:* Gierisch, Jennifer, et al. "The impact of wearable motion sensing technologies on physical activity: A systematic review." VA ESP Project 09–010 (2015).

57 *abandon them within six months*: Endeavor Partners. "The future of activity trackers (part 3): The secret to long-term engagement." (2014).

57 *get step counts right*: Evenson, Kelly, Michelle Goto, and Robert Furberg. "Systematic review of the validity and reliability of consumer-wearable activity trackers." *International Journal of Behavioral Nutrition and Physical Activity* 12.1 (2015): 1–22.

57 *the same goes for smartphone apps:* Case, Meredith, et al. "Accuracy of smartphone applications and wearable devices for tracking physical activity data." *JAMA* 313.6 (2015): 625–626.

57 *study of four popular devices:* Nelson, Benjamin, et al. "Validity of consumer-based physical activity monitors for specific activity types." *Medicine & Science in Sports & Exercise* 48.8 (2016): 1619–1628.

57 *readings for cycling and weight lifting:* Nelson, Benjamin, et al. "Validity of consumer-based physical activity monitors for specific activity types." *Medicine & Science in Sports & Exercise* 48.8 (2016): 1619–1628; Bai, Yang, et al. "Comparison of consumer

and research monitors under semistructured settings." *Medicine & Science in Sports & Exercise* 48.1 (2016): 151–158.

58 *surveys show:* Kay, Melissa, et al. "Awareness and knowledge of the 2008 Physical Activity Guidelines for Americans." *Journal of Physical Activity & Health* 11.4 (2014): 693–698.

58 *what research shows:* Tudor-Locke, Catrine, et al. "Revisiting 'how many steps are enough?'" *Medicine & Science in Sports & Exercise* 40.7 (2008): S537–S543; Tudor-Locke, Catrine, et al. "How many steps/day are enough? for adults." *International Journal of Behavioral Nutrition and Physical Activity* 8 (2011): 79.

58 *study of people who had osteoarthritis:* White, Daniel, et al. "Walking to meet physical activity guidelines in knee osteoarthritis: Is 10,000 steps enough?" *Archives of Physical Medicine and Rehabilitation* 94.4 (2013): 711–717.

CHAPTER 5

67 *researchers have found this method to be lacking:* Sarzynski, Mark, et al. "Measured maximal heart rates compared to commonly used age-based prediction equations in the Heritage Family Study." *American Journal of Human Biology* 25.5 (2013): 695–701.

69 *heat-regulating system becomes more efficient:* Lee, Jeong-Beom, et al. "Long distance runners present upregulated sweating responses than sedentary counterparts." *PloS One* 9.4 (2014): e93976.

70 *regimen developed by Martin Gibala:* Gibala, Martin, et al. "Physiological adaptations to low-volume, high-intensity interval training in health and disease." *Journal of Physiology* 590.5 (2012): 1077–1084.

70 *HIIT training known as Tabata:* Tabata, Izumi, et al. "Effects of moderate-intensity endurance and high-intensity intermittent training on anaerobic capacity and VO2." *Medicine & Science in Sports & Exercise* 28.10 (1996): 1327–1330.

70 *7-Minute Workout:* Klika, Brett, and Chris Jordan. "High-intensity circuit training using body weight: Maximum results with minimal investment." *ACSM's Health & Fitness Journal* 17.3 (2013): 8–13; Reynolds, Gretchen. "The scientific 7-minute workout." *New York Times* May 9 (2013).

71 *HIIT increases VO2 max:* Milanović, Zoran, Goran Sporiš, and Matthew Weston. "Effectiveness of high-intensity interval training (HIT) and continuous endurance training for VO2max improvements: A systematic review and meta-analysis of controlled trials." *Sports Medicine* 45.10 (2015): 1469–1481.

71 *HIIT can improve:* Kessler, Holly, Susan Sisson, and Kevin Short. "The potential for high-intensity interval training to reduce cardiometabolic disease risk." *Sports Medicine* 42.6 (2012): 489–509; Ramos, Joyce, et al. "The impact of high-intensity interval training versus moderate-intensity continuous training on vascular function: A systematic review and meta-analysis." *Sports Medicine* 45.5 (2015): 679–692.

71 *reducing so-called subcutaneous fat:* Boutcher, Stephen. "High-intensity intermittent exercise and fat loss." *Journal of Obesity* (2011): 868305.

71 *study by Japanese researchers:* Nemoto, Ken-ichi, et al. "Effects of high-intensity interval walking training on physical fitness and blood pressure in middle-aged and older people." *Mayo Clinic Proceedings* 82.7 (2007): 803–811.

71 *review of 10 studies:* Weston, Kassi, Ulrik Wisløff, and Jeff Coombes. "High-intensity interval training in patients with lifestyle-induced cardiometabolic disease: A systematic review and meta-analysis." *British Journal of Sports Medicine* 48.16 (2014): 1227–1234.

71 *people who have type 2 diabetes:* Jelleyman, Charlotte, et al. "The effects of high-intensity interval training on glucose regulation and insulin resistance: A meta-analysis." *Obesity Reviews* 16.11 (2015): 942–961.

71 *it's generally safe:* Levinger, Itamar, et al. "What doesn't kill you makes you fitter: A systematic review of high-intensity interval exercise for patients with cardiovascular and metabolic diseases." *Clinical Medicine Insights: Cardiology* 9 (2015): 53–63.

72 *study by Martin Gibala:* Gillen, Jenna, et al. "Twelve weeks of sprint interval training improves indices of cardiometabolic health similar to traditional endurance training despite a five-fold lower exercise volume and time commitment." *PloS One* 11.4 (2016): e0154075.

72 *research in young, physically active women:* McRae, Gill, et al. "Extremely low volume, whole-body aerobic–resistance training improves aerobic fitness and muscular endurance in females." *Applied Physiology, Nutrition, and Metabolism* 37.6 (2012): 1124–1131.

72 *people react negatively:* Saanijoki, Tiina, et al. "Affective responses to repeated sessions of high-intensity interval training." *Medicine & Science in Sports & Exercise* 47.12 (2015): 2604–2611.

72 *study of 44 inactive adults:* Jung, Mary, Jessica Bourne, and Jonathan Little. "Where does HIT fit? An examination of the affective response to high-intensity intervals in comparison to continuous moderate- and continuous vigorous-intensity exercise in the exercise intensity-affect continuum." *PloS One* 9.12 (2014): e114541.

72 *study of subjects who were unfit:* Kilpatrick, Marcus, et al. "Impact of high-intensity interval duration on perceived exertion." *Medicine & Science in Sports & Exercise* 47.5 (2015): 1038–1045.

73 *people with prediabetes:* Jung, Mary, et al. "High-intensity interval training as an efficacious alternative to moderate-intensity continuous training for adults with prediabetes." *Journal of Diabetes Research* (2015): 191595.

73 *HERITAGE Family Study:* Skinner, James, et al. "Age, sex, race, initial fitness, and response to training: The HERITAGE Family Study." *Journal of Applied Physiology* 90.5 (2001): 1770–1776.; Bouchard, Claude, et al. "Familial aggregation of VO2 max response to exercise training: Results from the HERITAGE Family Study." *Journal of Applied Physiology* 87.3 (1999): 1003–1008.

73 *By the researchers' estimates:* Bouchard, Claude, et al. "Familial aggregation of VO2 max response to exercise training: Results from the HERITAGE Family Study." *Journal of Applied Physiology* 87.3 (1999): 1003–1008.

74 *four-week trial:* Schoenfeld, Brad Jon, et al. "Body composition changes associated with fasted versus non-fasted aerobic exercise." *Journal of the International Society of Sports Nutrition* 11.1 (2014): 54.

74 *study involving overweight women:* Gillen, Jenna, et al. "Interval training in the fed or fasted state improves body composition and muscle oxidative capacity in overweight women." *Obesity* 21.11 (2013): 2249–2255.

74 *adaptations that could in theory enhance performance:* Van Proeyen, Karen, et al. "Beneficial metabolic adaptations due to endurance exercise training in the fasted state." *Journal of Applied Physiology* 110.1 (2011): 236–245.

CHAPTER 6

77 *health benefits of strength training:* Westcott, Wayne. "Resistance training is medicine: Effects of strength training on health." *Current Sports Medicine Reports* 11.4 (2012): 209–216.

79 *help decrease body fat:* Strasser, Barbara, and Wolfgang Schobersberger. "Evidence for resistance training as a treatment therapy in obesity." *Journal of Obesity* (2011): 482564.

79 *aerobic exercise is more effective:* Vissers, Dirk, et al. "The effect of exercise on visceral adipose tissue in overweight adults: A systematic review and meta-analysis." *PloS One* 8.2 (2013): e56415.

79 *combination of resistance and aerobic training:* Ho, Suleen, et al. "The effect of 12 weeks of aerobic, resistance or combination exercise training on cardiovascular risk factors in the overweight and obese in a randomized trial." *BMC Public Health* 12 (2012): 704.

80 *doing more reps:* Garber, Carol Ewing, et al. "American College of Sports Medicine position stand. Quantity and quality of exercise for developing and maintaining cardiorespiratory, musculoskeletal, and neuromotor fitness in apparently healthy adults: Guidance for prescribing exercise." *Medicine & Science in Sports & Exercise* 43.7 (2011): 1334–1359.

80 *doing fewer reps:* Schoenfeld, Brad, et al. "Muscular adaptations in low-versus high-load resistance training: A meta-analysis." *European Journal of Sport Science* 16.1 (2016): 1–10.

80 *number of reps and the size of the weight generally don't matter:* Morton, Robert, et al. "Neither load nor systemic hormones determine resistance training-mediated hypertrophy or strength gains in resistance-trained young men." *Journal of Applied Physiology* 121.1 (2016): 129–138.

80 *research shows that this can enhance results:* Rhea, Matthew, and Brandon Al-

derman. "A meta-analysis of periodized versus nonperiodized strength and power training programs." *Research Quarterly for Exercise and Sport* 75.4 (2004): 413–422.

81 *BFR appears to increase muscle size:* Slysz, Joshua, Jack Stultz, and Jamie Burr. "The efficacy of blood flow restricted exercise: A systematic review & meta-analysis." *Journal of Science and Medicine in Sport* 19.8 (2016): 669–675.

81 *BFR has potential risks:* Scott, Brendan, et al. "Exercise with blood flow restriction: An updated evidence-based approach for enhanced muscular development." *Sports Medicine* 45.3 (2015): 313–325.

82 *approach can produce superior strength gains:* Westcott, Wayne, et al. "Effects of regular and slow speed resistance training on muscle strength." *Journal of Sports Medicine and Physical Fitness* 41.2 (2001): 154–158.

82 *several trials in older people:* Reid, Kieran, and Roger Fielding. "Skeletal muscle power: a critical determinant of physical functioning in older adults." *Exercise and Sport Sciences Reviews* 40.1 (2012): 4–12.

82 *beneficial for maintaining and building bone:* Zhao, Renqing, Meihua Zhao, and Liuji Zhang. "Efficiency of jumping exercise in improving bone mineral density among premenopausal women: A meta-analysis." *Sports Medicine* 44.10 (2014): 1393–1402.

84 *core exercises can relieve low-back pain:* Chang, Wen-Dien, Hung-Yu Lin, and Ping-Tung Lai. "Core strength training for patients with chronic low back pain." *Journal of Physical Therapy Science* 27.3 (2015): 619–622.

84 *evidence they can improve physical functioning:* Granacher, Urs, et al. "The importance of trunk muscle strength for balance, functional performance, and fall prevention in seniors: A systematic review." *Sports Medicine* 43.7 (2013): 627–641.

84 *study of fit men in their 20s:* Alcaraz, Pedro, et al. "Similarity in adaptations to high-resistance circuit vs. traditional strength training in resistance-trained men." *Journal of Strength and Conditioning Research* 25.9 (2011): 2519–2527.

84 *follow-up trial:* Romero-Arenas, Salvador, et al. "Effects of high-resistance circuit training in an elderly population." *Experimental Gerontology* 48.3 (2013): 334–340.

85 *American Council on Exercise commissioned a study:* Stenger, Edward, et al. "Abs abs abs." American Council on Exercise (2014).

85 Consumer Reports *study:* "The coaster is not all that clear." *Consumer Reports* September (2010).

86 *studies show can be effective:* Loveless, Melinda, and Joseph Ihm. "Resistance exercise: How much is enough?" *Current Sports Medicine Reports* 14.3 (2015): 221–226.

87 *may reduce the effectiveness of strength training:* Panissa, Valéria, et al. "Acute effect of high-intensity aerobic exercise performed on treadmill and cycle ergometer on strength performance." *Journal of Strength and Conditioning Research* 29.4 (2015): 1077–1082.

87 *researchers assigned physically active young men*: Schumann, Moritz, et al. "Fitness and lean mass increases during combined training independent of loading order." *Medicine & Science in Sports & Exercise*, 46.9 (2014): 1758–1768.

87 *12-week study involving older men:* Wilhelm, Eurico Nestor, et al. "Concurrent strength and endurance training exercise sequence does not affect neuromuscular adaptations in older men." *Experimental Gerontology* 60 (2014): 207–214.

88 *beginners experience strength gains more rapidly:* Kraemer, William, and Nicholas Ratamess. "Fundamentals of resistance training: Progression and exercise prescription." *Medicine & Science in Sports & Exercise* 36.4 (2004): 674–688.

CHAPTER 7

90 *study of 1,400 runners:* Pereles, Daniel, Alan Roth, and Darby Thompson. "A large, randomized, prospective study of the impact of a pre-run stretch on the risk of injury on teenage and older runners." USA Track & Field (2010).

91 *echoed by other trials:* Small, Katie, Lars McNaughton, and Martyn Matthews. "A systematic review into the efficacy of static stretching as part of a warm-up for the prevention of exercise-related injury." *Research in Sports Medicine* 16.3 (2008): 213–231.

91 *evidence for this isn't ironclad:* McHugh, Malachy, and Ciaran Cosgrave. "To stretch or not to stretch: The role of stretching in injury prevention and performance." *Scandinavian Journal of Medicine & Science in Sports* 20.2 (2010): 169–181.

91 *review of randomized studies:* Herbert, Robert, Marcos de Noronha, and Steven Kamper. "Stretching to prevent or reduce muscle soreness after exercise." *Cochrane Database Systematic Reviews* 7 (2011): CD004577.

91 *one of the reviewed studies:* Jamtvedt, Gro, et al. "A pragmatic randomised trial of stretching before and after physical activity to prevent injury and soreness." *British Journal of Sports Medicine* 44.14 (2010): 1002–1009.

91 *review of more than 100 studies:* Simic, Luka, Nejc Sarabon, and Goran Markovic. "Does pre-exercise static stretching inhibit maximal muscular performance? A meta-analytical review." *Scandinavian Journal of Medicine & Science in Sports* 23.2 (2013): 131–148.

92 *two reviews of studies:* Cheatham, Scott, et al. "The effects of self-myofascial release using a foam roll or roller massager on joint range of motion, muscle recovery, and performance: A systematic review." *International Journal of Sports Physical Therapy* 10.6 (2015): 827–838; Schroeder, Allison, and Thomas Best. "Is self myofascial release an effective preexercise and recovery strategy? A literature review." *Current Sports Medicine Reports* 14.3 (2015): 200–208.

92 *combining SMR with static stretching:* Mohr, Andrew, Blaine Long, and Carla Goad. "Effect of foam rolling and static stretching on passive hip-flexion range of motion." *Journal of Sport Rehabilitation* 23.4 (2014): 296–299.

92 *may reduce soreness:* Cheatham, Scott, et al. "The effects of self-myofascial re-

lease using a foam roll or roller massager on joint range of motion, muscle recovery, and performance: A systematic review." *International Journal of Sports Physical Therapy* 10.6 (2015): 827–838.

92 *technique may even improve it:* MacDonald, Graham, et al. "Foam rolling as a recovery tool after an intense bout of physical activity." *Medicine & Science in Sports & Exercise* 46.1 (2014): 131–142.

93 *less research on PNF stretching:* Behm, David, et al. "Acute effects of muscle stretching on physical performance, range of motion, and injury incidence in healthy active individuals: A systematic review." *Applied Physiology, Nutrition, and Metabolism* 41.1 (2015): 1–11.

93 *odd finding in some research:* Cramer, Joel, et al. "The acute effects of static stretching on peak torque, mean power output, electromyography, and mechanomyography." *European Journal of Applied Physiology* 93.5–6 (2005): 530–539.

93 *study of young and middle-aged men:* Behm, David, et al. "Relative static stretch-induced impairments and dynamic stretch-induced enhancements are similar in young and middle-aged men." *Applied Physiology, Nutrition, and Metabolism* 36.6 (2011): 790–797.

93 *study involving female high school athletes:* Chatzopoulos, Dimitris, et al. "Acute effects of static and dynamic stretching on balance, agility, reaction time and movement time." *Journal of Sports Science & Medicine* 13.2 (2014): 403–409.

94 *study of golfers:* Moran, Kieran, et al. "Dynamic stretching and golf swing performance." *International Journal of Sports Medicine* 30.2 (2009): 113–118.

94 *short static stretches are less likely to impair performance:* Behm, David, and Anis Chaouachi. "A review of the acute effects of static and dynamic stretching on performance." *European Journal of Applied Physiology* 111.11 (2011): 2633–2651.

94 *you may experience greater improvements:* Garber, Carol Ewing, et al. "American College of Sports Medicine position stand. Quantity and quality of exercise for developing and maintaining cardiorespiratory, musculoskeletal, and neuromotor fitness in apparently healthy adults: Guidance for prescribing exercise." *Medicine & Science in Sports & Exercise* 43.7 (2011): 1334–1359.

96 *increase flexibility in as little as four weeks:* Cipriani, Daniel, et al. "Effect of stretch frequency and sex on the rate of gain and rate of loss in muscle flexibility during a hamstring-stretching program: A randomized single-blind longitudinal study." *Journal of Strength and Conditioning Research* 26.8 (2012): 2119–2129; de Baranda, Pilar Sainz, and Francisco Ayala. "Chronic flexibility improvement after 12 week of stretching program utilizing the ACSM recommendations: Hamstring flexibility." *International Journal of Sports Medicine* 31.6 (2010): 389–396.

96 *stretch at least three days a week:* Garber, Carol Ewing, et al. "American College of Sports Medicine position stand. Quantity and quality of exercise for developing and maintaining cardiorespiratory, musculoskeletal, and neuromotor fitness in apparently healthy adults: Guidance for prescribing exercise." *Medicine & Science in Sports & Exercise* 43.7 (2011): 1334–1359.

96 *Starting around age 30 or 40*: de Oliveira Medeiros, Hugo Baptista, et al. "Age-re-lated mobility loss is joint-specific: An analysis from 6,000 Flexitest results." *Age* 35.6 (2013): 2399–2407.

96 *shoulders and trunk tend to lose flexibility more quickly*: de Oliveira Medeiros, Hugo Baptista, et al. "Age-related mobility loss is joint-specific: An analysis from 6,000 Flexitest results." *Age* 35.6 (2013): 2399–2407.

96 *vary from one side to another:* Soucie, Michael, et al. "Range of motion measure-ments: Reference values and a database for comparison studies." *Haemophilia* 17.3 (2011): 500–507.

96 *sports-related injuries:* Baeza-Velasco, Carolina, et al. "Joint hypermobility and sport: A review of advantages and disadvantages." *Current Sports Medicine Reports* 12.5 (2013): 291–295.

96 *risk of anxiety disorders:* Baeza-Velasco, Carolina, et al. "Joint hypermobility and sport: A review of advantages and disadvantages." *Current Sports Medicine Reports* 12.5 (2013): 291–295.

97 *survey of hot yoga practitioners:* Mace, Casey, and Brandon Eggleston. "Self-re-ported benefits and adverse outcomes of hot yoga participation." *International Jour-nal of Yoga Therapy* 26.1 (2016): 49–53.

97 *stretching muscles that are heated:* Nakano, Jiro, et al. "The effect of heat applied with stretch to increase range of motion: A systematic review." *Physical Therapy in Sport* 13.3 (2012): 180–188.

99 *tool to predict mortality risk:* de Brito, Leonardo Barbosa Barreto, et al. "Ability to sit and rise from the floor as a predictor of all-cause mortality." *European Journal of Preventive Cardiology* 21.7 (2014): 892–898.

99 *indicator of flexibility:* Brito, Leonardo Barbosa Barreto, Denise Sardinha Mendes Soares de Araújo, and Claudio Gil Soares de Araújo. "Does flexibility influence the ability to sit and rise from the floor?" *American Journal of Physical Medicine & Reha-bilitation* 92.3 (2013): 241–247.

CHAPTER 8

104 *many experts believe is too low:* Rodriguez, Nancy, and Sharon Miller. "Effective translation of current dietary guidance: Understanding and communicating the con-cepts of minimal and optimal levels of dietary protein." *American Journal of Clinical Nutrition* 101.6 (2015): 1353S–1358S.

104 *levels are not thought to cause harm:* Phillips, Stuart, Daniel Moore, and Jason Tang. "A critical examination of dietary protein requirements, benefits, and excesses in athletes." *International Journal of Sport Nutrition and Exercise Metabolism* 17 (2007): S58–S76.

104 *Goldilocks amount:* Thomas, Travis, Kelly Anne Erdman, and Louise Burke. "Po-sition of the Academy of Nutrition and Dietetics, Dietitians of Canada, and the Amer-

ican College of Sports Medicine: Nutrition and athletic performance." *Journal of the Academy of Nutrition and Dietetics* 116.3 (2016): 501–528.

104 *around .9 grams per pound:* Thomas, Travis, Kelly Anne Erdman, and Louise Burke. "Position of the Academy of Nutrition and Dietetics, Dietitians of Canada, and the American College of Sports Medicine: Nutrition and athletic performance." *Journal of the Academy of Nutrition and Dietetics* 116.3 (2016): 501–528.

104 *trying to maximize gains in strength:* Cermak, Naomi, et al. "Protein supplementation augments the adaptive response of skeletal muscle to resistance-type exercise training: A meta-analysis." *American Journal of Clinical Nutrition* 96.6 (2012): 1454–1464.

104 *exercise vigorously while on a low-calorie diet:* Longland, Thomas, et al. "Higher compared with lower dietary protein during an energy deficit combined with intense exercise promotes greater lean mass gain and fat mass loss: A randomized trial." *American Journal of Clinical Nutrition* 103.3 (2016): 738–746.

104 *eating 20 or 30 grams of protein:* Areta, José, et al. "Timing and distribution of protein ingestion during prolonged recovery from resistance exercise alters myofibrillar protein synthesis." *Journal of Physiology* 591.9 (2013): 2319–2331; Symons, Brock, et al. "A moderate serving of high-quality protein maximally stimulates skeletal muscle protein synthesis in young and elderly subjects." *Journal of the American Dietetic Association* 109.9 (2009): 1582–1586.

104 *research on this is mixed:* Aragon, Alan, and Brad Schoenfeld. "Nutrient timing revisited: Is there a post-exercise anabolic window." *Journal of the International Society of Sports Nutrition* 10.1 (2013): 5.

104 *science is even less conclusive:* Beck, Kathryn, et al. "Role of nutrition in performance enhancement and postexercise recovery." *Open Access Journal of Sports Medicine* 6 (2015): 259–267.

105 *eating up to seven a week*: Rong, Ying, et al. "Egg consumption and risk of coronary heart disease and stroke: Dose-response meta-analysis of prospective cohort studies." *BMJ* 346 (2012): e8539.

106 *research as a whole has failed to prove:* Messina, Mark. "Soybean isoflavone exposure does not have feminizing effects on men: A critical examination of the clinical evidence." *Fertility and Sterility* 93.7 (2010): 2095–2104.

106 *may adversely affect thyroid levels:* Messina, Mark, and Geoffrey Redmond. "Effects of soy protein and soybean isoflavones on thyroid function in healthy adults and hypothyroid patients: A review of the relevant literature." *Thyroid* 16.3 (2006): 249–258.

107 *carbs may help endurance athletes:* Moore, Daniel. "Nutrition to support recovery from endurance exercise: Optimal carbohydrate and protein replacement." *Current Sports Medicine Reports* 14.4 (2015): 294–300.

107 *chocolate milk:* Pritchett, Kelly, and Robert Pritchett. "Chocolate milk: A post-exercise recovery beverage for endurance sports." *Medicine and Sport Science* 59 (2012): 127–134.

107 *influenced by makers of sports beverages:* Cohen, Deborah. "The truth about sports drinks." *BMJ* 345 (2012): e4737.

107 *most people typically get enough water:* Panel on Dietary Reference Intakes for Electrolytes and Water. *Dietary Reference Intakes for Water, Potassium, Sodium, Chloride, and Sulfate.* National Academies Press (2005).

108 *studies involving competitive cyclists:* Goulet, Eric. "Effect of exercise-induced dehydration on time-trial exercise performance: A meta-analysis." *British Journal of Sports Medicine* 45.14 (2011): 1149–1156.

108 *advice on many websites*: Hoffman, Martin, Theodore Bross III, and Tyler Hamilton. "Are we being drowned by overhydration advice on the Internet?" *Physician and Sportsmedicine* 44.4 (2016): 343–348.

108 *not generally a cause of muscle cramps:* Braulick, Kyle, et al. "Significant and serious dehydration does not affect skeletal muscle cramp threshold frequency." *British Journal of Sports Medicine* 47.11 (2013): 710–714; Hoffman, Martin, and Kristin Stuempfle. "Muscle cramping during a 161-km ultramarathon: Comparison of characteristics of those with and without cramping." *Sports Medicine-Open* 1 (2015): 24; Nolte, Heinrich, et al. "Exercise-associated hyponatremic encephalopathy and exertional heatstroke in a soldier: High rates of fluid intake during exercise caused rather than prevented a fatal outcome." *Physician and Sportsmedicine* 43.1 (2015): 93–98.

108 *report authored by a panel of 17 experts:* Hew-Butler, Tamara, et al. "Statement of the third international exercise-associated hyponatremia consensus development conference, Carlsbad, California, 2015." *Clinical Journal of Sport Medicine* 25.4 (2015): 303–320.

110 *researchers peed all over the notion:* Heneghan, Carl, et al. "Mythbusting sports and exercise products." *BMJ* 345 (2012): e4848.

110 *creatine can increase muscle mass and strength:* Devries, Michaela, and Stuart Phillips. "Creatine supplementation during resistance training in older adults—a meta-analysis." *Medicine & Science in Sports & Exercise* 46.6 (2014): 1194–1203.

110 *improve performance at high-intensity exercises:* Cooper, Robert, et al. "Creatine supplementation with specific view to exercise/sports performance: An update." *Journal of the International Society of Sports Nutrition* 9.1 (2012): 33.

111 *caffeine can improve performance in endurance activities:* Ganio, Matthew, et al. "Effect of caffeine on sport-specific endurance performance: A systematic review." *Journal of Strength and Conditioning Research* 23.1 (2009): 315–324.

111 *boost for high-intensity exercises:* Astorino, Todd, and Daniel Roberson. "Efficacy of acute caffeine ingestion for short-term high-intensity exercise performance: A systematic review." *Journal of Strength and Conditioning Research* 24.1 (2010): 257–265.

111 *can provide an exercise boost:* Higgins, Simon, Chad Straight, and Richard Lewis. "The effects of pre-exercise caffeinated-coffee ingestion on endurance performance: An evidence-based review." *International Journal of Sport Nutrition and Exercise Metabolism* 26.3 (2016): 221–239.

REFERENCES

111 *energy drinks and shots*: Rosenbloom, Christine. "Energy drinks, caffeine, and athletes." *Nutrition Today* 49.2 (2014): 49–54.

112 *linked to the deaths:* Food and Drug Administration, "FDA consumer advice on pure powdered caffeine." fda.gov December (2015).

112 *increase heart rate and decrease blood flow:* Higgins, John, and Kavita Babu. "Caffeine reduces myocardial blood flow during exercise." *American Journal of Medicine* 126.8 (2013): 730.e1–730.e8.

112 *beta alanine supplements may improve performance:* Hobson, Ruth, et al. "Effects of β-alanine supplementation on exercise performance: A meta-analysis." *Amino Acids* 43.1 (2012): 25–37.

112 *activity lasting one to four minutes:* Trexler, Eric, et al. "International Society of Sports Nutrition position stand: Beta-alanine." *Journal of the International Society of Sports Nutrition* 12.1 (2015): 1–14.

112 *healthy people in their 70s, 80s, and even 90s:* Stout, Jeffrey, et al. "The effect of beta-alanine supplementation on neuromuscular fatigue in elderly (55–92 years): A double-blind randomized study." *Journal of the International Society of Sports Nutrition* 5.1 (2008): 1–6; del Favero, Serena, et al. "Beta-alanine (Carnosyn™) supplementation in elderly subjects (60–80 years): effects on muscle carnosine content and physical capacity." *Amino Acids* 43.1 (2012): 49–56; McCormack, William, et al. "Oral nutritional supplement fortified with beta-alanine improves physical working capacity in older adults: A randomized, placebo-controlled study." *Experimental Gerontology* 48.9 (2013): 933–939.

112 *compound in muscles called carnosine:* Blancquaert, Laura, Inge Everaert, and Wim Derave. "Beta-alanine supplementation, muscle carnosine and exercise performance." *Current Opinion in Clinical Nutrition & Metabolic Care* 18.1 (2015): 63–70.

113 *may decrease muscle soreness:* da Luz, Claudia, et al. "Potential therapeutic effects of branched-chain amino acids supplementation on resistance exercise-based muscle damage in humans." *Journal of the International Society of Sports Nutrition* 8 (2011): 23.

113 *haven't been shown to improve athletic performance*: Negro, Massimo, et al. "Branched-chain amino acid supplementation does not enhance athletic performance but affects muscle recovery and the immune system." *Journal of Sports Medicine and Physical Fitness* 48.3 (2008): 347–351.

113 *little science to support their use;* Gunnels, Trint, and Richard Bloomer. "Increasing circulating testosterone: Impact of herbal dietary supplements." *Journal of Plant Biochemistry & Physiology* 2.2 (2014): 130; Qureshi, Ahmed, Declan Naughton, and Andrea Petroczi. "A systematic review on the herbal extract tribulus terrestris and the roots of its putative aphrodisiac and performance enhancing effect." *Journal of Dietary Supplements* 11.1 (2014): 64–79; Willoughby, Darryn, Mike Spillane, and Neil Schwarz. "Heavy resistance training and supplementation with the alleged testosterone booster NMDA has no effect on body composition, muscle performance, and serum hormones associated with the hypothalamo-pituitary-gonadal axis in resistance-trained males." *Journal of Sports Science & Medicine* 13.1 (2014): 192–199;

Wilborn, Colin, et al. "Effects of zinc magnesium aspartate (ZMA) supplementation on training adaptations and markers of anabolism and catabolism." *Journal of the International Society of Sports Nutrition* 1.2 (2004): 12–20.

113 *reports of serious side effects:* Food and Drug Administration, "Public health advisory: The FDA recommends that consumers should not use body building products marketed as containing steroids or steroid-like substances." fda.gov July (2009).

115 *research has failed to show:* Peternelj, Tina-Tinkara, and Jeff Coombes. "Antioxidant supplementation during exercise training." *Sports Medicine* 41.12 (2011): 1043–1069.

115 *may even block some of the benefits of exercise:* Paulsen, Goran, et al. "Vitamin C and E supplementation alters protein signalling after a strength training session, but not muscle growth during 10 weeks of training." *Journal of Physiology* 592.24 (2014): 5391–5408; Bjørnsen, Thomas, et al. "Vitamin C and E supplementation blunts increases in total lean body mass in elderly men after strength training." *Scandinavian Journal of Medicine & Science in Sports* 26.7 (2016): 755–763.

115 *"at the least, useless":* Gomez-Cabrera, Mari Carmen, Michael Ristow, and Jose Viña. "Antioxidant supplements in exercise: Worse than useless?" *American Journal of Physiology-Endocrinology and Metabolism* 302.4 (2012): E476–E477.

115 *beneficial for overall health*: Carlsen, Monica, et al. "The total antioxidant content of more than 3100 foods, beverages, spices, herbs and supplements used worldwide." *Nutrition Journal* 9 (2010): 3

116 *people are more likely to overeat them:* Suher, Jacob, Raj Raghunathan, and Wayne Hoyer, "Eating healthy or feeling empty? How the "healthy = less filling" intuition influences satiety." *Journal of the Association for Consumer Research* 1.1 (2016): 26–40.

116 *branded as "fitness" foods:* Koenigstorfer, Joerg, and Hans Baumgartner. "The effect of fitness branding on restrained eaters' food consumption and post-consumption physical activity." *Journal of Marketing Research* 53.1 (2016): 124–138.

CHAPTER 9

121 *review of 17 trials:* Bleakley, Chris, et al. "Cold-water immersion (cryotherapy) for preventing and treating muscle soreness after exercise." *Cochrane Database of Systematic Reviews* 2 (2012): CD008262.

121 *ideally for 10 to 15 minutes*: Machado, Aryane Flauzino, et al. "Can water temperature and immersion time influence the effect of cold water immersion on muscle soreness? A systematic review and meta-analysis." *Sports Medicine* 46.4 (2016): 503–514.

121 *review of four studies:* Costello, Joseph, et al. "Whole-body cryotherapy (extreme cold air exposure) for preventing and treating muscle soreness after exercise in adults." *Cochrane Database of Systematic Reviews* 9 (2015): CD010789.

121 *head-to-head comparison:* Petrofsky, Jerrold, et al. "Cold vs. heat after exercise—

is there a clear winner for muscle soreness." *Journal of Strength and Conditioning Research* 29.11 (2015): 3245–3252.

121 *pooling data from 13 studies:* Bieuzen, François, Chris Bleakley, and Joseph Thomas Costello. "Contrast water therapy and exercise induced muscle damage: A systematic review and meta-analysis." *PLoS One* 8.4 (2013): e62356.

121 *review of nine studies:* Torres, Rui, et al. "Evidence of the physiotherapeutic interventions used currently after exercise-induced muscle damage: Systematic review and meta-analysis." *Physical Therapy in Sport* 13.2 (2012): 101–114.

122 *some studies refute this idea:* Nelson, Nicole. "Delayed onset muscle soreness: Is massage effective?" *Journal of Bodywork and Movement Therapies* 17.4 (2013): 475–482; Wiltshire, Victoria, et al. "Massage impairs postexercise muscle blood flow and 'lactic acid' removal." *Medicine & Science in Sports & Exercise* 42.6 (2010): 1062–1071.

123 *research by and large has failed to prove:* Vella, Luke, et al. "Ibuprofen ingestion does not affect markers of post-exercise muscle inflammation." *Frontiers in Physiology* 7 (2016): 86.

123 *participants in the Western States Endurance Run:* Nieman, David, et al. "Ibuprofen use, endotoxemia, inflammation, and plasma cytokines during ultramarathon competition." *Brain, Behavior, and Immunity* 20.6 (2006): 578–584.

123 *may aggravate the problem:* Van Wijck, Kim, et al. "Aggravation of exercise-induced intestinal injury by Ibuprofen in athletes." *Medicine & Science in Sports & Exercise* 44.12 (2012): 2257–2262.

123 *studies in rodents support this idea:* Schoenfeld, Brad. "The use of nonsteroidal anti-inflammatory drugs for exercise-induced muscle damage: Implications for skeletal muscle development." *Sports Medicine* 42.12 (2012): 1017–1028.

123 *several studies in humans:* Schoenfeld, Brad. "The use of nonsteroidal anti-inflammatory drugs for exercise-induced muscle damage: Implications for skeletal muscle development." *Sports Medicine* 42.12 (2012): 1017–1028.

123 *little evidence that it reduces DOMS:* Barlas, Panos, et al. "Managing delayed-onset muscle soreness: Lack of effect of selected oral systemic analgesics." *Archives of Physical Medicine and Rehabilitation* 81.7 (2000): 966–972.

124 *small, randomized study:* Connolly, Declan, et al. "Efficacy of a tart cherry juice blend in preventing the symptoms of muscle damage." *British Journal of Sports Medicine* 40.8 (2006): 679–683.

124 *study not funded by industry:* Bell, Phillip, et al. "The effects of Montmorency tart cherry concentrate supplementation on recovery following prolonged, intermittent exercise." *Nutrients* 8.7 (2016): 441.

124 *research involving marathon runners and cyclists:* Howatson, Glyn, et al. "Influence of tart cherry juice on indices of recovery following marathon running." *Scandinavian Journal of Medicine & Science in Sports* 20.6 (2010): 843–852; Bell, Phillip, et al. "Recovery facilitation with Montmorency cherries following high-intensity,

metabolically challenging exercise." *Applied Physiology, Nutrition, and Metabolism* 40.4 (2014): 414–423.

124 *research in rats*: Tall, Jill, et al. "Tart cherry anthocyanins suppress inflammation-induced pain behavior in rat." *Behavioural Brain Research* 153.1 (2004): 181–188.

125 *may provide short-term relief:* Cao, Huijuan, et al. "Cupping therapy for acute and chronic pain management: A systematic review of randomized clinical trials." *Journal of Traditional Chinese Medical Sciences* 1.1 (2014): 49–61.

125 *most of the studies are of poor quality:* Cao, Huijuan, et al. "An overview of systematic reviews of clinical evidence for cupping therapy." *Journal of Traditional Chinese Medical Sciences* 2.1 (2015): 3–10; Kim, Jong-In, et al. "Cupping for treating pain: A systematic review." *Evidence-Based Complementary and Alternative Medicine* (2011): 467014.

126 *fear of injury is a common barrier*: Centers for Disease Control and Prevention, "Overcoming barriers to physical activity." cdc.gov; Canadian Fitness and Lifestyle Research Institute. Physical Activity Monitor. (1995).

126 *injury rates of older people:* Little, Robert, et al. "A 12-month incidence of exercise-related injuries in previously sedentary community-dwelling older adults following an exercise intervention." *BMJ Open* 3.6 (2013): e002831.

126 *decrease your chances of getting injured:* Campbell, Kristin, et al. "Injuries in sedentary individuals enrolled in a 12-month, randomized, controlled, exercise trial." *Journal of Physical Activity & Health* 9.2 (2012): 198–207.

129 *Army recruits who smoked:* Altarac, Maja, et al. "Cigarette smoking and exercise-related injuries among young men and women." *American Journal of Preventive Medicine* 18.3S (2000): 96–102.

129 *Other research in military recruits:* Heir, Trond, and G. Eide. "Injury proneness in infantry conscripts undergoing a physical training programme: Smokeless tobacco use, higher age, and low levels of physical fitness are risk factors." *Scandinavian Journal of Medicine & Science in Sports* 7.5 (1997): 304–311.

129 *research in teenage athletes:* Milewski, Matthew, et al. "Chronic lack of sleep is associated with increased sports injuries in adolescent athletes." *Journal of Pediatric Orthopaedics* 34.2 (2014): 129–133.

129 *weight lifters wind up in U.S.emergency rooms:* Kerr, Zachary, Christy Collins, and Dawn Comstock. "Epidemiology of weight training-related injuries presenting to United States emergency departments, 1990 to 2007." *American Journal of Sports Medicine* 38.4 (2010): 765–771.

130 *study that followed long-distance runners ages 50 and older:* Chakravarty, Eliza., et al. "Long distance running and knee osteoarthritis: A prospective study." *American Journal of Preventive Medicine* 35.2 (2008): 133–138.

130 *surveyed former college swimmers*: Sohn, Roger, and Lyle Micheli. "The effect of running on the pathogenesis of osteoarthritis of the hips and knees." *Clinical Orthopaedics and Related Research* 198 (1985): 106–109.

REFERENCES

130 *runners have a* lower *risk of joint problems:* Cymet, Tyler Childs, and Vladimir Sinkov. "Does long-distance running cause osteoarthritis?" *Journal of the American Osteopathic Association* 106.6 (2006): 342–345.

131 *evidence supporting the practice isn't ironclad:* Collins, Niamh. "Is ice right? Does cryotherapy improve outcome for acute soft tissue injury?" *Emergency Medicine Journal* 25.2 (2008): 65–68.

REFERENCES

INDEX

INDEX

224